The Weight of Happiness

On Food, Body and Spirit

The Weight of Happiness

On Food, Body, and Spirit

Ayelet Kalter

The poem **The Fat Sumo Man** by Yona Wallach in the opening of the book was published in its original Hebrew version in the book **Sub-consciousness Opens Like a Fan**, Hakibbutz Hameuhad Publishing, Simanei Kriah Books, 1992.

The rights to the quote from the book **Love's Executioner: And Other Tales of Psychotherapy** by Irvin D. Yalom belong to Basic Books Inc. Publishers, New York, 1989.

The poem **How Does the Man Look Who's Right** by Adam Zagajewski was published in English in the collection, **Without End**, Farrar, Straus & Giroux, New York, 2002.

Contact: ayelet@eatingdialog.com
Website: www.eatingdialog.com
www.healthypeoplecomeinallsizes.com

ISBN-13: 978-1540386045
ISBN-10: 154038604X

To Tamar

The Fat Sumo Man

Has handcuffs on

When I speak to you

I see you from all the distances

This Fat Sumo Man

Is the true criminal

What did he really do

I have forgotten what

But something wrong

You can feel

This man

Is everything I

Don't allow myself

He is all about propriety so to speak

He is all about absence of freedom

He is all about restraint

But you can say the opposite

He is all about freedom

He is all about forbidden lusts

But he is truly

All the anguishes.

Yona Wallach

Foreword

No, I am not fat, and this book is not the outcome of years of suffering from frustrating diets.

Nor do I attempt to bring you the "ultimate diet."

Though I have never suffered from being overweight, I am plagued by the epidemic of slimness and figure, and like many of us, am preoccupied with my body in a rather obsessive manner.

My family has a prominent history of being overweight, and I distinctly remember instances at home when we spoke about the need to be careful and not gain weight. I even recall myself at the ages of seven and eight standing with my protruding belly and my mother telling me, "Stand up straight and tuck your tummy."

I remember very well the iron rules in our home concerning food, and the fear we felt that if we didn't watch it, we would gain weight, and if we weren't strict, we would become fat.

I don't exactly know why, but despite my genetics, I am a woman of normal body weight today. Perhaps there was something in the habits and awareness of eating that I attained that has helped me maintain a comfortable, healthy body weight.

It is important for me to maintain a body weight that doesn't weigh me down or encumber my movements. It is important for me to feel at ease with my body. And this is what I believe in for everyone.

Hence, the road to studying nutrition and dieting seemed natural, but it would be too presumptuous or insincere to tie the two together. I actually began my studies at the agriculture faculty where I studied animals, but I took a year off to travel to the Far East. Upon my return, I changed my course of study on a whim, and I found myself discovering the world of clinical nutrition.

On completing my studies as a dietician, I slowly became privy to the world of obesity in all its complexities.

From my work in the field, I soon realized that diet—as a food plan in the purely conventional sense of the word—cannot really answer the needs of my patients.

Moreover, I recognized that the professional skills and abilities I have acquired in my studies were insufficient in dealing with the painful and vexing world of obesity. It is a world in which more is there than meets the eye.

One of the cases that had a profound effect on me early on in my career was the story of three siblings in a family that I treated.

It was during the Pentecost Jewish festival.[1] They took turns talking about the food their mother had prepared and

---

[1]Also known as *Shavuot* in Hebrew, or Feast of Weeks in English, this Jewish holiday occurs on the sixth day of the Hebrew month of Sivan, marking the all-important wheat harvest in the Land of Israel, and commemorates the anniversary of the day God gave the Torah to the entire nation of Israel assembled at Mount Sinai.

the quantities. I had a hard time imagining and grasping what was being said. But then the youngest brother said he had eaten dumplings, the middle brother—forty, and the eldest brother—sixty. I asked,

"How many did your mother prepare?" And when they replied with a round number of 200, I felt my entire world of reference had just crumbled. With mustered strength, I managed to stop my face from grimacing in astonishment.

And so, little by little, I began to understand that for many people, days of heavy caloric intake are simply routine and are not necessarily viewed as binges or loss of control.

For instance, a patient's daily report:

- Breakfast—two slices of bread with Munster cheese and a cup of coffee
- In between—Croissant with ice-blended coffee
- Fixed lunch menu: Salad with blue cheese and walnuts broiled fish with baked potato, glass of wine
- Afternoon—Ice cream bar for a snack
- Dinner—A plate of hummus with two pitas
- Night—Grapes, two peaches, two plums

Calories: 4,000. No binges or loss of control, but a lot of food.

Other people do experience binges. A binge may include two chocolate bars, a chocolate chip ice cream container, 200 grams (7 oz.) of nuts and a pack of butter-drenched cookies, and the hand (or rather the mouth) still outstretched.

And so through my patients, I took my first steps in the enigmatic, concealed world of eating. I learned that nothing is predictable. That not all overeating is a binge, and not all overeating ends in thousands of calories.

I realized that people have a hard time sharing what happens among themselves, and more so, about food. I realized that from the moment a person is caught in the vicious cycle of eating, he is at times completely disconnected from himself and his environment, drowning in a stupor whose degree of damage he may only fathom later on.

Only a few of the binges occur in a sober state of mind, in a fleeting moment of self-destruction.

Most of them involve fatigue, guilt, anger, self-loathing and a sense of worthlessness.

The hardest thing for a person is to discuss his binge when his biggest wish is to quickly forget everything, hide the event, and remove all evidence from himself and his surroundings. But the evidence remains, as a silent testimony, in the burdening excess weight.

At the end of each session, I would be left with my patients' pain, their frustration over the difficulty to cope, and mainly with my own frustration over my inability to truly help them. I would try to brainstorm with them about where exactly they felt stuck. What caused this stagnation? What did they think could help them? I would try to come up with different, varied food plans to enliven the faltering process of losing weight.

I would try to encourage and console every time they regained all the weight they had lost. Many times, I found myself in a "therapeutic merry-go-round" that went around and around but never really accomplished much: the patient struggled to lose weight and, even more so, to maintain the loss. And I stood helpless before him, unable to help, and finding it hard to contain both his and my own disappointment.

Back then, I didn't dare speak about giving up the unrealized "fantasy of slimness." I still believed that one could help people reach fictional goal weights and become thin.

I had yet to understand that helping a patient did not necessarily mean he would lose all the weight he believed was in excess, which was the reason for most of his problems — the chip on his shoulder.

I didn't understand nor dare to admit to myself that perhaps not everyone was meant to be "thin." And that many people can be happy and lead a full life without being slim.

It gradually sank in that the solution, if one can even use that term, is not in another food plan or another dieting regime. I realized that a therapeutic goal could help a person discover what and where the healthy, right place is for him. This place doesn't have to be measured by his ability to achieve the ideal weight on a numbered scale.

I began to feel that I had to deepen and develop my therapeutic tools and not just rely on the knowledge I had acquired in the world of calories and food combinations.

I tried to understand the motives, hardship, frustration, dilemmas, and most of all, the pain that accompanied the weight of people who came to me for help.

I felt that calorie deficit wasn't enough to enable weight loss and that weight loss wasn't something that could be simply controlled by will power. I realized that self-control and abstinence are not enough to solve the countless problems hiding beneath that excess weight.

And so I tried, and still do, to acquire new tools that would enable me to help my patients, who are walking the tightrope connecting body and spirit.

In the following lines, I shall try to give you a glimpse into the intricate world of knowledge accumulated over the years around the treatment of obesity.

Obesity is perceived to be a result of a complex, dynamic interaction between physiological, psychological, social, cultural and ecological factors.

"Overweight" is the term for excess weight above a desired weight range according to sex, age and height. It can stem from the accumulation of fat and from added muscle mass resulting from intense physical exercise.

"Obesity," however, refers to excess weight beyond the range, due to a discrepancy between a person's energy consumption and energy exertion.

Being that with most people, their excess weight is the result of excess fat, I shall discuss excess weight as overweight.

Overweight is defined as a weight that is 20 percent above the ideal body weight, or a BMI (Body Mass Index) of over 25.

Today, the simplest, most common method to measure weight gain is the BMI, which denotes the ratio between the body weight and height of a healthy adult. It serves as an easy, preliminary tool to determine the state of one's weight. Its disadvantage lies in the fact that it doesn't take into consideration age, sex and body type, and in many cases does not serve as an accurate index for fat mass and its distribution in the body. It is calculated as the body weight (in kilograms [Kg.]) divided by the square of the body height (in meters.)

For example, if a person is 1.65 meters high (5'4") and weighs 55 Kg. (121 Lbs.), his BMI is 20.2.

The BMI scale is:
20–25 healthy weight
25–30 overweight
30–35 obese
35–40 severely obese
Above 40, we are talking about morbidly obese.

Therefore, slimming means losing weight according to these values.

It is important to remember that:

1. In recent years, obesity has gradually become a global epidemic bearing heavy medical, financial and social consequences.
2. Obesity has become a complex problem, resistant to treatment. Nearly 95 percent of the people who lose weight gain it back, sometimes with surplus, within five years.

What is it about obesity that makes it so resistant to treatment and so painful and frustrating? What is it that, despite all the health complications involved and social codes of beauty and slimness, most people find hard to battle?

Perhaps it would be fair to examine the world of obesity from a systematic perspective.

From a cultural-social standpoint, there is no doubt that the "slimness ideal" plays an important part in how obesity is viewed. For years, the pursuit of slimness has spurred the development of a frustrating and painful "dieting" culture, which, absurdly, goes hand in hand with exacerbating the obesity problem. If dieting was once synonymous with a nutritional eating plan of a medical nature, the word diet is now synonymous with an entire industry.

The human body has a control system that regulates food consumption and energy exertion so that both a person's body and his physical constitution are maintained. This system governs the amount of consumed energy and its composition.

According to the Set Point Theory, every person has his typical body weight, which is partially a hereditary trait determined by the brain. Fluctuations in body weight under or over the individual's point of equilibrium will stimulate the central nervous system to activate the appetite and metabolism to protect the Set Point.

While one can challenge this point with rigorous physical exercise and a strict caloric reduction, as soon as those are ceased, the weight will climb back up to the equilibrium point.

In order to try to conform to social pressure and the slimness culture, many fat people are in a constant state of real hunger and lack of energy, since they are desperately trying to keep their body weight below the Set Point. Hence, many people who lose weight are placed in biological underweight. They are trapped in an impossible position, within a system of pressures that are applied to them from two directions. On the one hand, there are social and health pressures to lose weight, and on the other, is the body's biological resistance to fluctuations in weight. And they are stuck in the middle.

Thus, the system that regulates the energy balance in the body arouses a strong urge to eat after a significant weight loss in order to maintain stability. This fact obviously makes it hard for those trying to maintain the weight loss.

Research on families and twins shows that the genetic aspect has great influence on the development of obesity.[2] But while many are willing to accept the fact that genetic factors contribute, for instance, to a difference in height among people, they find it hard to accept the differences in weight.

Just like there are genetic differences, perhaps there are also differences in our basic urges. And perhaps, the fat person has a strong, burning need for control when he must resist the urge to eat, and that need increases after he has lost some weight. And perhaps, the more he loses weight, the more he feels hungry, and this hunger is much stronger than his conscious desire to be thin.

That increased hunger is indicated by recent studies having found higher levels of Gherlin, "the hunger hormone,"[3] among people who have lost weight by dieting, compared to the hormone levels prior to dieting.

---

[2]The research was conducted by Dr. Albert J. Stunkard, a leading psychiatrist in the field of eating disorders at the University of Pennsylvania.

[3]Leidy, H. J. J. K. Gardner, B.R. Frye, M.L. Snook, M. K. Schuchert, E. L. Richard and N.I. Williams, "Circulating Gherlin Is Sensitive to Changes in Body Weight During a Diet and Exercise Program in Normal-Weight Young Women," *The Journal of Clinical Endocrinology & Metabolism*, (June 2004), 89 (6), p. 2659-2664.

Hence, it may be inferred that losing weight is a battle against natural, innate powers and the urge to eat is often internal and cannot be changed.

Aside from biological mechanisms, eating is also influenced by the environment, whether through aggressive advertising channels or exposure to an endless variety of appetizing food products.

We are governed to a considerable degree by cognitive aspects that affect our eating behaviors. Many of our daily activities are influenced by external signals in our day-to-day routines such as bedtime, waking time, etc. These signals set conditioned times that drive us to eat.

Senses such as smell, sight, taste and touch have an effect on arousing hunger. Some are dictated by cultural customs and some by each person's cravings and desires. We are driven to satisfy cravings for unique flavors of sweet, sour, salty and bitter, and even the color of the food affects us.

Eating is a basic, vital survival action, primarily motivated by an existential, physiological need. Often, the boundary between the physiological role of food and eating and other roles—big or small—projected onto it gets blurred.

Food, handling it, dieting and even weight gain often play emotional roles. Sometimes, these roles are so deeply rooted that the person finds it hard to disengage from the support that food provides for him, finding it difficult to live without these alternatives.

In daily life, we often fall into using food as a means, a tool to desensitize an emotion (anxiety), express an emotion (love), handle an emotion, and sometimes simply to not feel. As early as 1957, Kaplan viewed overeating as an acquired response to reducing anxiety.[4]

According to researchers, overweight people find it hard to discern between hunger and anxiety, since they are used to eating as a response to fear just as they are used to eating in response to hunger.

There is something intimidating about connecting and feeling painful emotions such as loneliness and sexuality. Food can prevent such emotion from surfacing in our consciousness. And if an emotion does come up, food can numb it and cover it up. Gorging on large quantities can numb an emotion to the point where it is no longer felt.

Writers belonging to the psychoanalytic approach have expanded the dialogue further by assuming that overeating is the result of inner conflicts between the id, the ego, and the superego.

The id is the container of impulsive energy, the dwelling place of the impulses for life and death. It serves as the person's source of spiritual energy and is beyond the individual's awareness.

Ego is the personality's foreign minister—the authority responsible for the personality's contact with reality.

The superego is the minister of morality, possessing all the cultural and social values and norms that determine the

---

[4]Kaplan, H., Kaplan, H.S. 1957. "The psychosomatic concept of obesity," *Journal of Nervous and Mental Disease.*

rules of conduct pertaining to prohibitions and limitations on the one hand and aspirations on the other.

There is a constant interplay between these three entities, since they are interdependent in forming any action taken by that personality.

According to Freud, founder of the psychoanalytic approach, sexual impulses are prominent in all stages of life.[5] In each stage, a few defense mechanisms are formed to prevent a person from being aware of his instincts and sexual impulses, which have been frustrated and unsatisfied in full. Conflict arises in the struggle between the different entities. When the conflict is not resolved well, symptoms may develop. On this basis, one can see how gaining weight and overeating is a symptom of unresolved conflict.

Hamburger, for example, viewed obesity as a fixation of the oral stage. A stage in which the child is breastfed with his mother's milk and forms a link between receiving love and being fed. Such a fixation in this stage is the outcome of either lacking or overindulging in motherly love. Later on, when these people have increased oral demands and the need for warmth and love is not properly satisfied, eating replaces them due to the unconscious link between food and love.[6]

Even the British psychoanalyst D.W. Winnicott pointed to a similar way of thinking in which food becomes a means, a

---

[5]"Sexuality and The Psychology of Love," Sigmund Freud, Philip Rieff, Simon and Schuster, Apr 1, 1997
[6]Walter W. Hamburger, Med Clinic, North Am. 1951 Mar; 35(2):483–499.
[7]"Playing and Reality," D.W. Winnicott, 1971, Tavistock Publications Ltd.

tool that blends the physical and emotional experience at the onset of our life.[7] He spoke often about the unique connection between the motherly figure and the baby, one that creates a strong bond between food, warmth, love, and security. And then, during adulthood when we feel emotional deprivation, we naturally return to those familiar, known sensations and try to recreate them. Since our experience of eating brings up feelings of warmth, love, and comfort, we feed ourselves in order to relive those sensations.

Some researchers tend to view obesity as a fixation that begins during the anal stage. In this stage, the child seeks independence and self-expression, while his parents try to teach him hygiene habits and conformism. Overeating is a compulsive habit of hoarding, through which a person expresses resistance toward anyone who tries to determine or guide his behavior.

Many people find it hard to be mindful and identify the hunger signals inside them, relying mainly on external signals in order to stop and/or encourage eating. Such external signals may be a smell, opportunities to eat such as dining at a restaurant, certain times, the look and color of the food, etc.

Some researchers assume that there is a system of physiological hunger signals that include stomach contractions, which they believe are learned. Some people have internalized them while others have not. Those who have not rely more on external signals as eating stimulants and tend to overeat.

For example, stomach contractions decrease during stress, which cause some people to cut down on their eating. Those who do not interpret the contractions as hunger signals will not cut down on their eating since they are not attuned to such signals.

Hence, we hear of people who eat more when they are anxious, while others feel blocked and completely satisfied.

Some believe that people who are overweight have experienced a disruption in the experiential, interpersonal process that involves the gratification of needs.[8] They believe that obesity is the use of food in response to signs of emotional tension on the one hand and a failure to respond by eating when truly hungry on the other. Thus, eating becomes a frequent response to any strong emotional state. This acquired response leads to improper eating habits and makes it hard for many people to feel and know when they are hungry and when they are satiated. They need external signals to know when to eat and how much since their self-awareness and consciousness have not been adequately programmed.

The balance between the desire to eat on the one hand and the effort to avoid it by resistance and restraint of that urge on the other, have a profound effect on eating behaviors. The restraint is a cognitive effort of resistance and

---

[8]Hilda Baruch, a psychoanalyst who has dealt with eating disorders extensively.
[9]"Dietary restraint: A theoretical and empirical review" by Ruderman, Audrey J. *Psychological Bulletin*, Vol 99(2), Mar 1986, 247-262.

abstinence. People who forcefully restrain their eating are almost always in a state of constant worry about what they will eat, when, and how much, for fear of gaining weight. The main problem is that this powerful and extreme control over eating is disrupted once in a while by events that call for lack of control (i.e., the Restraint Hypothesis.[9]) Such situations may include a distorted perception of eating by increasing the quantities. So if a person who is dieting and feels like he must eat according to a set plan deviates in quantities of foods that are "not allowed" (such as pizza, chocolate...) or perceived by him as "forbidden," he feels himself a failure. And, from an outlook of "all or nothing," he loses control over the food and goes into binges, whose underlying basis is one of guilt, shame, and unworthiness.

Situations such as smoking marijuana or highly charged emotional states such as anxiety and depression may trigger an uncontrollable binge among those people under restriction, who practice restraint and abstinence.

The idea behind this theory is that, among people who restrain their eating, emotional states, having their self-esteem threatened or endangered triggers increased eating up to bouts of binging.

Some people find it hard or impossible to rely on other people to fulfill their "others but myself" needs, and instead of turning to people, they turn to food to fulfill these needs.

Heinz Kohut, a psychoanalyst and founder of the "Self"[10] psychology, claims in his theory that the self is the

[10]*Heinz Kohut (Psychanalystes d'aujourd'hui)*, Published January 1st 1998 by Presses Universitaires de France

individual's psychological center of the universe, to which we refer by saying: "I feel so and so," "I do so and so." The healthy human self is experienced as a feeling of wholeness, vitality, and strength. The inner needs of the self to which we relate are the need for self-value, regulation of emotions, calmness and security, vitality, and a feeling of continuity over time and space.

According to Kohut, the term "others but myself" refers to experiencing the other person as functioning in a way that supports our self.[11]

Kohut claims that every healthy person needs his inner needs fulfilled, at least in part, by others. However, he views relying on "others but myself" as flexible, and an unhealthy self is highly dependent on others to do for him what his own self cannot. This is where food fills a role in that person's life. Food is so concrete that it serves as emotional crutches for many people, an alternative for others but themselves, which they have difficulty finding.

Often, the food, eating, and preoccupation with dieting simply serve as a veil meant to shift the focus from the real problem. The more a person is preoccupied with food, calories, and cycles of gaining and losing weight, the more he falls into the tempting web of a purely concrete preoccupation while removing himself from the real difficulties. As much as the obsession with dieting and the losing-gaining cycles are

---

[11]Bachar, Dr. Eytan. *The Fear of Occupying Space*. Magnus Publishing, 2000.

painful, it enables a person to engage in something concrete, something that defines the emotions and feelings that may seem unsolvable.

A person can engage in binging, purging, control the types of food he eats and the quantities, and— All but the real issues are hidden beneath them. That person has a hard time telling the concrete from the symbolic. He finds it hard to see in the concrete something that represents things like pain, difficulty in interpersonal relationships, and unresolved conflicts.

When a person sinks into the convoluted world of eating, he succeeds for certain lengths of time, to descend into a subconscious realm that numbs the true feelings that he finds hard to contain. For example, the experience of a binge is perceived by many as being in a trance. Similar feelings of being high and euphoria are brought on by fasting.

People who are addicted to diets and binges alternately often find themselves in a cycle of addiction that is hard to come out of, especially because it plays a role in that person's life. As made up as it may sound, that person has a hard time connecting to his body and feelings, and due to his inability to contain the pain involved, he sinks into a cycle of dieting and binging. That person's strong desire to control his feelings and life end up controlling him.

Considering this theory, we must try to understand women, their feelings, and their behavior toward their body against the backdrop of Western culture, politics, and philosophy. Obesity represents a deliberate—aware or unaware—affront against sexually and culturally defined stereotypes. As such, we can view fat as related to protection, sex, endowment, power, boundaries, motherly care, decisiveness, and anger.[12]

Thus, food gradually becomes a tool. It can be used as an alibi to avoid social interactions and intimacy, which often can be threatening for fear of rejection.

For many people, food is a communication tool for feelings and thoughts that they find hard to express. So, for example, if a child finds it hard to set boundaries for his parents who are invading his privacy and his life, he will do so by eating or not eating, as if saying, "I control my body, here you can't decide for me or control me."

Many people are afraid to touch and feel, so in order to keep a safe distance from their emotions and bodies, they distract themselves by engaging in food thoughts and activities. Just so they won't allow themselves to feel.

And there is a difference between feelings and behavior.

Behavior can be controlled. Feelings cannot.

If we ignore our feelings, they will intensify, and their expression may be destructive or perverted. When we stop treating our emotions as the enemy, we can perhaps develop a different relationship with them.

And since we have different emotions, we cannot respond to every emotion in the same way—by eating.

We cannot:

- Feel angry, and eat.
- Feel sad and eat.

---

[12]Susie Orbach, one of the most famous psychologists and feminist critics in the world, who has been fighting the slimness tyranny for years.

- Feel anxious and eat.
- Feel happy and eat.

Hunger for food, as said, is an existential need, a survival necessity. But eating is not always driven purely out of need to satisfy the body. Sometimes, it is driven by a need for pleasure, social gathering, or religious ritual. In most of these cases, the decision and choice to eat is with the person.

But sometimes, a person finds himself unable to control his eating, feeling as if his eating is dictated by a power outside of his control during intense emotional states or when overpowered by strong, uncontrollable desires.

Sometimes, this leads to an obsessive preoccupation with food, accompanied by feelings of guilt and loss of control over eating behaviors. Such people do not experience themselves as having the choice or ability to know what, when and how much to eat. They are governed by beliefs and myths, by aggressive marketing and advertising methods, by new diets that appear on the scene every other day, and by the slimness ideal that is rooted in our culture, bringing frustration and agony to many, due to its unattainability.

Many of these people suffer from binge eating, a phrase first coined in 1950 by Stunkard.[13]

A binge is the effect of eating and the mood, rather than merely the amount of food consumed. A person may

---

[13]The research was conducted by Dr. Albert J. Stunkard, a leading psychiatrist in the field of eating disorders at the University of Pennsylvania.

experience binge eating even when few calories are consumed. This experience usually has a few characteristics:

- Emotionally, the binge usually begins with a sense of pleasure derived from the food, but gradually turns into feelings of disgust by what accompanies the eating and its consequences.
- The pace of eating. Most binges are characterized by fast consumption that may reach 81.5 calories a minute, versus normal eating of 38.4 calories a minute.
- A sense of excitement and thrill during the eating that most people describe as a sense of ecstasy, like taking drugs or being in a trance.
- Secrecy, eating in hiding.
- Loss of control over eating.[14]

These binges are part of an endless cycle moving between dieting and binging. This cycle involves harsh dieting, low self-esteem, obsessive preoccupation with body and weight, and heavy emotional distress within a person. All of these may trigger binge eating. After such eating, a person feels guilty and desperate, which leads to a bad mood and low self-esteem, which once again triggers the desire for harsh dieting or alternatively a strong desire to eat. Thus, a person enters a vicious, frustrating and painful cycle.

---

[14]Christopher G. Fairburn, *Overcoming Binge Eating*. The Guilford Press, 1995. Dr. Fairburn is a leading psychiatrist from Oxford University who specializes in obesity and eating disorders and is developing a cognitive-behavioral approach to handling them.

All around us, millions of people have just ended a diet or are searching for the "ultimate diet." Their lives revolve in a vicious cycle of losing and gaining weight. Moreover, some will increase their weight from one diet to the next. Yet most people never give up the euphoric feeling of a "dieting success" nor the humiliation and failure that follow.

The belief that life will change if and when weight is lost is also an inseparable aspect of their life. For many, this is an alibi. Meaning, in their perception, everything will be different when they lose weight. All will change. As long as they are not losing, nothing can really change. Everything is stuck.

"It's all the weight's fault."

"When we lose weight, we can have a proper relationship."

"When we lose weight, we can try changing jobs."

"When we lose weight, we'll be happier."

In fact, some people put their entire lives on hold, in a holding pattern, to reach a better place with their body weight. They believe that only when they are truly thin, things can change. And, naturally, if such a person "slips" and eats say a slice of pizza, he immediately deems himself a reckless sinner, a complete failure, because his is an "all or nothing" approach. He launches a wild eating binge, because all is lost, and he is left with enduring pain and suffering.

And the same goes for the scale.

Many people set their day according to what number they read on the scale. And if the scale shows a number that does not fit in with their self-perception, it immediately becomes dominant and decisive. A person is no longer rational, blaming himself with countless negative emotions and self-deprecation for having a weak character and no will power. He experiences himself as a total failure, and this will determine how he feels and behaves that day. A person tends to humiliate and punish himself in response to his self-criticism, often without real grounds, but simply based on erroneous perceptions and unrealistic expectations of himself. Some people will hide at home and avoid social activities to the extent of skipping work or daily commitments.

Until not long ago, eating disorders and obesity have mainly been a problem among women. In recent years, the problem has spread and eaten away at men, too.

Still, the majority of those seeking treatment are women, and most women are engaged in dieting and worrying about their weight. Many women find themselves having a futile, painful eating dialogue with their bodies, their eating behaviors, and the food they choose or do not choose to eat. And, indeed, the stories I chose to bring to you involve women.

I chose to look at the world of obesity and eating problems through their intricate personal prism and as part of a social fabric.

The society we live in is a competitive, goal-oriented and extroverted one, which has muddled all the social stereotypes of the past and left the woman confronted with numerous roles, torn between her commitments to society, family and to herself.

The female body has always been shaped and suited to fulfill society's expectations. It has undergone changes judged by men and women. During the Victorian age, the ideal of feminine beauty was a fleshy woman, shaped like an hourglass. Women wore restrictive corsets to accentuate their narrow waists and show off their rear, which caused many digestive and respiratory problems.

Internalizing the value of beauty and slimness began in the 1920s, when the flat look became popular. Women tied their breasts to attain the side view of an ironing board. After World War I, another change came about whereby body fat was perceived as inefficient and a sign of self-indulgence.

The new style emphasized slim figures and narrow waists. Women viewed this style as a symbol of freedom and liberation. But, against the freedom from corsets and cumbersome dresses, an enslavement to dieting began to take place. The idea that the body could be controlled and shaped by practicing self-control became the guideline of social perception.

Another change occurred during that period. Modernization and the industrial era brought along the manufacturing of set sizes. Women found themselves measured according to the size of the clothes manufactured, and whoever did not fit into those limitations learned the hard way that her body did not fit the norm.

In the fifties, a thin woman with large breasts was considered attractive, and the voluptuous Marilyn Monroe set a new standard. But in the sixties, things changed again, and the emaciated slimness in the image of Twiggy became a major symbol of physical attraction. The emphasis on weight loss was intensified.

And today?

Women have to be thin, but not altogether fragile. Dieting is not enough; physical exercise is also compulsory. The goal is to reach the impossible ideal of a thin, starved body, sculpted and slim—with big breasts, of course.

And the woman?

She has become a slave to her body.

Her body has become a battlefield.

We should also consider the complexity of a woman's countless roles in the modern world.

She has become independent and freer financially and personally.

The external changes of socioeconomic, sexual, and professional open-mindedness have created ambiguity in the definitions and essence of interpersonal relationships. The internalization process of these changes has been slower and more complex than it seems, and is not up to par with the rapid social changes. This has led to an "internal splitting."

The equality between the sexes is far from being complete and real, and there is still sincere confusion between the roles that were once defined and clear.

Some say that the more women gain power and strength in their private, social, and financial life, the more they are demanded to appear scrawny, emaciated, inert and weak, as if seemingly lacking influence and unthreatening.

Thus, a woman is fighting an endless, weakening battle. A battle over her place in society, her place for herself, her body and her spirit.

Perhaps this book is part of that battle.

Preface

I invite you to join me on a journey that does not provide another solution or another weight loss program. I will not promise that you can achieve or maintain the dream of "ideal slimness."

I shall try to introduce you to a world in which weight, food, body, and spirit come together from a slightly different perspective. A world in which not everything has to be assessed by weight loss diets, weight, and calories; where success is a subjective place that causes a person to feel good about himself way beyond the kilograms, calories, and the number on the scale.

I shall do that by unfolding my therapeutic journey with a patient whose name in the book is Tamar.

Our journey lasted about two years and consisted of three major components.

A. Weekly sessions: In the short, half-hour sessions, the focus was on the cognitive and behavioral aspect of eating, as is reflected by the eating journals. In the longer, one-hour sessions, we addressed the emotional aspect underlying food.

B. Keeping a personal journal: Each of us documented our feelings, experiences, and discoveries from our own perspective. Tamar wrote about herself as a patient and the emotional processes she was undergoing, and I wrote about my feelings from my personal and professional perspective as the therapist.

C. Sessions that took place once in three months: These lasted a few hours and included reading all the material written in the time gaps between the sessions. Therefore, we also brought poems that we wrote to this session.

I am bringing forth the dialogue that took place between Tamar and me as-is, with no changes made.

Some short excerpts from other patients are incorporated into the journey with Tamar (under alias names as well). I believe the excerpts will shed light on some of the complexity surrounding the world of eating.

The book is printed in different fonts so as to distinguish between its three components.

It allows for a sensitive, at times painful, view into the boundless world underlying eating and weight gain. Perhaps this view will facilitate a different approach to looking at this world, and maybe even accepting it.

September 2000

You entered, looking down.

So did I.

I examined you from the corner of my eye as if I didn't know what you looked like.

A sagging shoulder, an embarrassed smile. You wore a white, somewhat elegant shirt with a maroon necklace and earrings. You had thick, wedged shoes on. You moved heavily toward the blue wicker chair in my office.

You sat down.

You were nervous.

So was I.

I shifted in my chair uneasily, trying to find a relaxed posture. As usual, I sat cross-legged on the seat of my chair, tilted my head forward, resting it in my left hand, fully there for you.

Tamar, you entered, enormous and amazing.

I sat behind a birch desk with heavy iron legs, painted in faded clouds of dirty white. There was a lot of blue around: in the paintings, the frames, the butterflies adorning them, and the sky peeking between the shutters. I have two mirrors in my office. One is long and narrow, hung opposite the patient's chair, so that when sitting opposite me, he can see himself from the corner of his eye. The second one is smaller and square and hangs above the scale. A few plants and plenty of quiet music. Hayden, Bach, Mozart.

And you here, Tamar.

With me.

Long legs, amazingly thin, a small, scrawny buttocks, and lots of stomach.

All here.

Between us two.

As with all first meetings, we both had expectations, fears, and anxiety all mixed up.

We began. A standard intake form full of technical details of age, personal status, family history, health condition, weight history, diet history, favorite foods, situations that trigger eating, physical activity, digestive function, addictions, smoking, sleeping habits, occupation, essentially any piece of information that could help me learn and put together the puzzle, even partially, of you and the environment surrounding you. I made sure to write everything down, even details I already knew.

The technical details:

Age forty-two.

Married with two children.

A warm, supportive home.

Works full-time. The director of an educational institution. Demanding job. Has been overweight for sixteen years, since her eldest daughter was born. Recalls herself with extra kilograms as early as elementary school, but it was always within the "normal" range for her. Esthetic and even sexy to some degree.

Like many others, she experienced the endless world of dieting from every possible angle. She is a graduate of failed attempts of "extreme dieting": acupuncture, fasting, diets according to eating plans or food groups, and the Weight Watchers' Points Plus diet. But despite the endless attempts, she still has an excess weight of 40 Kgs.

Health-wise she carries a long list of painful illnesses: unbalanced diabetes, high blood pressure, back problems, and cancer in remission.

Tamar's world is filled with activity. She works, volunteers in her community, and enriches herself with various cultural activities. Her days are full of interest and action, and eating is mainly focused on nighttime. She finds herself engaged in uncontrollable eating often. During the day, she also eats high-fat foods and large quantities.

She doesn't smoke, drink, or do any regular physical exercise, and is unable to drop the excess weight.

Height: 1.74 meters.

Therapeutic goal: losing weight to improve sugar levels and blood pressure, relieve the spine, and feel better in her body.

Standard protocol.

We shall try to infuse life into the treatment.

So far, Tamar, everything was familiar to you and even pretty standard. You expected a menu, a food plan. You waited for me to ask you how you eat, what you eat and when, so that together we could build a food plan for you. Perhaps more pleasant, friendlier, but still a food plan.

But I didn't pull out a food plan sheet or make a detailed list of what was allowed and what wasn't, what to eat, how much and when.

I tried to invite you on a somewhat different path.

I said to you,

"Tamar, I will not provide you with a written food plan or a calculated menu; a list of allowed and forbidden foods; an instruction of the total daily caloric intake; or a set of rules of what to eat, when and how much.

"I will provide you with pages. Pages in which you will try to track your eating behaviors. It allows for a slightly different journey, in which there are no structured meals, planned in advance, but a desire and attempt to understand your world of eating.

"Who is in control of it?

"What affects it?

"What do you choose to eat?

"Do you choose at all?

"Are you able to turn down food?

"Do you have any dialogue with your eating?

"What do you feel before you eat?

"What do you feel before and after eating?

"Are there instances when you eat and only later realize that you ate?

"Out of all this, perhaps we can create a change."

I watched you; you looked down. You seemed a little confused to me. This wasn't the plan you were waiting for, you said. In your mind, you imagined clear instructions for set meals.

But, no. No instructions. From now on, you choose and decide what to eat, if it's worth spending the calories, and what to spend them on. Whether you find it tasty.

"How will I know what's good and what's not?" you asked.

"How will I know that what I chose to eat is okay?"

"Tamar," I responded, "the amount of knowledge on food and diets you have accumulated over the years is immense. I believe that deep inside you, you know when you have gone too far, when you overeat, when you eat for no reason, and when you could have actually cut back a little. All I'm saying to you right now is try to think, prioritize, examine. Like in a clothing store. You enter the store, and there is a myriad of clothing in different colors and prices. Unfortunately, you can't buy everything due to sizes and money. You have to choose what is best for yourself and what you like the most. The same goes for food. You obviously can't eat everything because of the diabetes and the calories. And, just like excessive spontaneous shopping can lead to an overdraft, so does excessive eating cause weight gain. Therefore, you are not being judged or examined here, Tamar. You choose and ask only yourself. And if you feel good with your choices, then I will too."

I paused and watched your face. It was tense and concentrated. I continued:

"I know it's confusing. You feel rather lost, because when did you ever decide what to eat for yourself? You really only know two ways—either the dietician decides what you will eat or the food decides for you. But for you to decide for yourself?!

"I feel your concern, the uncertainty of what it would be like for you. How will you feel within this process? Where are you given the freedom of choice? Where are you told to decide? How can you best decide for yourself when you are not used to choosing?"

You looked at me, grimaced and said:
"Ayelet, it's different, strange. I don't know. I'm a little confused. I'm afraid I won't be able to track things consistently. I have never succeeded in a framework, let alone do homework? And besides, I have never managed my own food. It's a strange experience, which I don't know if I can go through. Also, do you think I can see for myself how much food I'm eating? I'll probably forget some of it. Do you know what happens there, with the food, the quantities?

"I'll be embarrassed to write them down, and even more so, show you...

"I understand your rationale. It resonates with me, it makes sense. But how will I be able to do that? I guess that if I track things, I will naturally eat less because I wouldn't want you to see what I'm eating and definitely not show it to you. But do you think it's so easy to simply eat less? And what if I don't succeed?"

I understood you, Tamar. Your fears, anxieties, dilemmas. I couldn't promise you anything. Only to try. I believed that if you would set off on your journey, things would change, things would happen.

"Tamar," I said, "I feel your concern and doubt, but at this stage, all I can tell you is let's try. Let's roll with it. We won't go too fast on this journey, and you can always stop at the closest station if you feel tired, overwhelmed or disappointed."

I sat silent.

You did too.

We sat staring at each other. In silence.

After a few minutes, you said:

"Ayelet, I think it's okay for me."

As for me? From the moment I got permission from you, I felt a rush of energy. I was eager to get started, and even more so, eager for you to succeed.

Like a turbo engine, I began to explain to you in further detail the rules of the game, the guidelines that would accompany us on our mutual journey.

I also tried to add a few small "requests" to the outline I laid out before you.

I asked that the food journal would be completely honest. Meaning that the journaling would be on the spot and as authentic as possible. "The pages are supposed to serve as a mirror," I said, "which you can look through and see reality as it truly is."

I asked that you would make sure the journaling is done the same day or even throughout the day so that there is no reliance on "selective memory" or ability to fix or change things. Because if the journaling is done after the fact, what good does it do?

I added, "And then, in each session, I will reflect to you what I see, what arises from the pages, the manner of eating, quantities, the type of food etc....through the pages, we will try to understand the nature of the eating and its motives. Tamar, I know that if you take even one tiny thing from everything I say in each session, internalize it, build one layer on top of another, a new and different perception of yourself and your eating will emerge. I hope that perhaps this way, you will develop a new set of beliefs and experiences that will enable you to act differently in your world of eating.

"The next rule I would like to provide you with, which may sound a little childish, is not to let others 'stick their nose' into your plate. It's important that you guard your privacy.

"Since the treatment we will undergo together has no allowed or forbidden foods, and since all food choices will be made by you only, it's important that you work on respecting your own choices, without others around you interfering, or saying:

"Is that allowed?"

"Is that written in your food plan?"

"How can you eat this while you're dieting?"

"Why are you paying your nutritionist so much if you can eat whatever you feel like?"

"Another important point is needing to have a daily plan. While every plan is subject to changes, your ability to plan out your day, Tamar, and how to fit the food into it, will contribute greatly to your success in better controlling your eating and being aware of it.

"For example, if you have a social dinner in a restaurant, what you have probably done up until now is not eat all day in order to use up all your food allowance at night, or you would eat before the event in order not to eat fatty foods with everyone else.

"In the first scenario, you show up 'starving,' which means your ability to control your eating is nearly impossible, and you eat anything and everything indiscriminately.

"In the second scenario, you watch everyone else in frustration, because they are all having a great time except for you. You just ate light bread at home while everyone else is indulging in a decent meal, in which case you either continuously eat out of frustration, because 'nothing matters' anyway or keep your frustration pent up until the late hours of the night and binge irrepressibly when you get home. You're angry at yourself, at the world, and at being deprived.

"I suggest you try to prepare differently for such an event, knowing that it's okay to enjoy it and eat there while trying to be economical at the same time. Meaning, show up with 'calories to spend' but not too hungry. Then, at the event, choose your favorite things and enjoy them with moderation.

"It sounds difficult, I know. But I believe that slowly but surely, with experience, you will begin to like these tools of planning and awareness. Perhaps they will improve your coping and choosing abilities. And maybe even your enjoyment.

"The last insight I would like to give you, Tamar, is the notion that we are not working on a project, but rather a process; a journey. And as such, it has a beginning, but the rest will be a result of the therapeutic relationship formed between us, of your needs, the type of journey we will undergo, its depth and its meaning for you."

I believe you remained silent through most of the session, Tamar. You listened, were surprised.

You didn't quite know how to walk this path. Will it be the right one for you?

How will you handle a framework that isn't really a framework?

How will you handle the fact that there is no dictated food plan? With the fact that nearly all the responsibility falls on you?

You didn't speak.

You looked at me, smiling shyly. Brushing away an unruly curl above a teary eye.

"Do we weigh you?" I asked.

You were caught off guard for a moment. You didn't know if you could look at the scale and see how much you weighed, and more so, that I would see. It didn't occur to you for one second that here you didn't have to be weighed, and that weighing is not a critical part of the agreement. You surely couldn't know that I don't even have to weigh someone in order to know how much they weigh.

What I see is enough.

What I feel is enough.

I left the choice to you.

I know it was a tough and anxious moment for you.

There is something about the numbers on the scale that arouse different fears and anger, which are sometimes hard to handle.

You looked at me as if expecting me to decide for you. I stared back, waiting, knowing that I must not interfere in these areas; they are yours.

A few moments of sweating and you decided to dare.

118.8 Kg. (261 Lbs.)

We began.

You left with blank paper and a few pointers that I tried to provide you.

I wondered if you were threatened by my attempts to invade, my desire to know what you eat, how much, why and when. Is it an intrusion on your secret world?

Did it feel right to you to be a partner in this journey?

And did my words resonate?

I knew I had to wait. Not nudge. Not proud. I had to be attuned to you, to your inner rhythm.

I was fearful for you as a patient and for me as a therapist.

But I was also hopeful.

***

I discovered you about eight years ago, Tamar, in a meditation workshop, just another gray afternoon in the fall.

You had this magnetizing magic about you.

I saw a powerful, sweeping, vibrant, large woman—fat.

A huge woman with a strong sense of presence about her.
And I, petite, slightly shy.

I say "discovered" because that is what it was—a discovery.
Masses of fat enveloping an incredible world of secrecy.

Inviting.

Burdening masses of fat, sliding down the slopes of life.

Cascading down.

The fate of brief encounters had our lives moving in
parallel lines with no significant intersecting points. A few
encounters in the occasional workshops, joint studies, all on
a banal, superficial level.

Incidental encounters, small talk and the occasional
"hello."

The change occurred at the entrance to the health clinic
I happened upon randomly, where I met you. It was an
ordinary morning, an ordinary encounter. When I asked
matter-of-factly, "How are you?"

"Sick, I guess."

"What?" I choked.

"Since when?"

"How come?"

"Cancer," you said. And that was enough.

I was dumbstruck.

As if possessed, from the depth of my terror and shock, I
asked, "I impose on you?"

And you so naturally said, "With pleasure."

"Impose?" That was the only word I could utter. I didn't
ask about help, visits, support. I said, "Impose."

And I started to impose. Full of fears and anxieties, for this illness is so intimidating, I imposed on you. I came every week, with a cake, a dish, a conversation and just my own self.

I wanted to be there for you, for myself.

Sometimes we spoke, sometimes you were weak, and sometimes Nadav would say that you needed quiet time.

I felt like my visits were welcomed. So I imposed on you some more and came. And you, you and Nadav, opened the door wide.

And I? I walked in.

And felt comfortable.

Despite the illness, the bald head, the suffering.

I saw you sick.

Up to your neck with an ailment that was threatening to swallow you.

That was also when I saw the fat. Cascading, yellowish, gooey.

I was angry at it, hated it; its size, its look, and mainly because it made you suffer.

Because aside from the cancer that raged in your body, you were afflicted with unregulated diabetes, high blood pressure and back problems. I knew well, what you have probably known for years: losing weight would not cure you, but losing 10 percent of your current weight would put you in a better place physically and emotionally, and could significantly relieve the ailments that had taken charge of your body and spirit.

So, I loathed it, the fat, and I so wanted it for you, but I didn't dare. Since when do I invite a patient to therapy? Since when do I initiate a session with a patient?

I kept watching silently.

A year went by. You got stronger. Slowly but surely, you came back to life. I watched you anxiously from the sidelines, your hair that started growing again, the rosiness that filled your cheeks again, your gradual return to work as well as to the heavier weight you started out with when the illness erupted (I think you added about 15 Kg. (33 Lbs.))

A year later, with many reservations, I found myself inviting you on a mutual journey.

It was at the end of Rosh Hashanah.[15]

The remains of the holiday sank into the fragrant, autumn night.

We sat in my backyard, soaking up the silence.

You and I.

"Tamar, this might seem intrusive, but I thought of suggesting we do something together about your body that is different than what you have probably done up until now. I'm not certain I can help you, but I thought we would try."

You looked at me, embarrassed, a little shocked. I invaded your privacy boldly without asking permission. I simply barged in. You shifted uncomfortably in the plastic chair, staring aimlessly at your toes and crushing the napkin between your fingers.

---

[15]The Jewish New Year.

You kept quiet for a moment.

You weren't mad, you didn't grimace. You were quiet.

I saw drops of sweat appear on your forehead, I felt your heart beating as you trembled slightly.

I did too.

"I don't know, I don't understand what it means, what it entails," you muttered. "I wasn't prepared for something like this."

"I know," I said.

And so, I invited you to join me in a process, a journey that would attempt to offer you a different way to handle the mounds of fat that overshadow your life. I thought that together we would try to approach your fat from different aspects that you had not yet touched on, and perhaps in this way, you could give up the vital role it plays in your life.

I felt that your fat covered up longings, needs, desires, frustration. I knew that dieting in its simplistic sense was deemed a total failure for you. Tamar, I knew that you were made up of so many layers, and under each layer hid a thicker one. But I thought that is what challenged me and aroused my curiosity. My wish to discover, know, and perhaps even bring relief and change.

I invited you to join me on a journey with a beginning. As for its end?

You looked at me, at once surprised and flattered.

"Why me?" you asked.

I didn't have a clear answer, it was more feelings, strong intuitions, nothing else that could promise you anything substantial.

I said, "Tamar, maybe together we can pave the road to a healthier place for you, where you will weigh a little less, eat healthy and feel better."

I told you I was inviting you on a path where we would get to know you and your hidden world beneath and behind the fat so that we could eventually bid farewell to at least some of the layers that burdened your body and spirit.

I didn't promise, I only invited.

"Let's gamble together," you said, "let's explore together. We will naturally gain something from the process, from the path."

And so, we embarked on this journey with no promises or expectations. We set out on a path we thought would teach us about each other.

I think it was the only thing we were clear about.

September 23, 2000

It's already Saturday, and only today, I managed to bring myself to meet myself.

A lot is going through my head, and everything is swept aside.

The choice is not to progress, to stay in the mundane.

There was excitement in Ayelet choosing me, and the same familiar feeling; people think there is something more to me until they know me better and find out there is nothing there. An empty space, dull, ordinary, full of fat, illnesses, food, pseudo-vibrant.

How long will it take her to find out and be disappointed?

But I was happy at the opportunity. Still not giving up on the vague desire to be lighter, healthier, and prettier and live a different life with my body.

I'm still not giving up.

We step toward each other cautiously.

Perhaps, this time,, something else will happen.

Maybe I will let her help me.

Maybe I could retreat to a less aware state, less complex, simple.

Like an infant.

Learning how to walk again in this mud. Not give off the old feeling that I have already tried it all, know it all. How can someone help me?

I'm an expert on destroying everything for myself inside and out, and I no longer care why.

I'm tired of it, I want to take care of myself, to breathe, build, make peace, find vitality. Not feel like I'm always apologizing for myself.

Maybe we will succeed in doing something?

It's good for me to track what I eat. I can see it's a lot. Enough for three people maybe, but I can't seem to eat less right now.

I find myself eating most of the day, mainly in the afternoon and evening. In the morning, during work, everything is sort of more organized. Two sandwiches that Nadav prepared for me, and if I stay late at work, I eat in the dining hall with the children and staff. But when I come back home at five in the afternoon, I'm hungry again, and I eat another full hot meal. In the evening, I have dinner with the kids, my own kids.

At night, I go to sleep at one or two in the morning, snacking in front of the TV up until then.

In fact, the moment I return home from work, I'm in one eating state or another. And there's always stuff to eat because I cook so well. It's a no-brainer. You cook whatever you lay your hands on and eat whatever you find.

I don't have any feelings of guilt nor a desire to eat less. I'm waiting for it to come from outside of me. I summon it with very little strength.

It doesn't come.

I know this thing has to be built from the inside. When will that momentum that I can never find come to me?

"Start each day anew," says Ayelet.

But I'm not even there.

Start a new what?

Every day, I binge anew. Besides, I don't have the ability to eat less right now, maybe just a little, for fear of the diabetes. I feel bad when the sugar goes up, and am afraid.

Ayelet.

Closed and ascetic, thin and depressed. Gathered to a tight pile of scrawny, skinny organs. Almost without body. The face of a young man mixed in with that of a woman's. High cheek bones aligned with a square, rigid chin. Thin creases frame thin lips, calculating words.

Blue eyes. Stainless steel diluted by a veil of tenderness. Almost without body, yet there, present, interesting. Like a poisonous snake swarm. Dangerous? So different from me.

Disciplined, punctual, organized and coherent. So opposed, yet doesn't arouse resistance in me. There is something melancholy and pleasant about her.

She is so different from my diffusions, my chaos, my fundamental lack of discipline. My inability to pick myself up and take action.

I have gone beyond the contempt I felt for myself for so many years. I'm screwing Mai and Ido up, my own kids. Mai is exactly like me, she craves good food. She enjoys everything

I cook. She tastes everything she sees. She can't be around food without wanting it.

And me, I comment, subjugate, frighten, threaten, "You'll end up looking like me."

On the one hand, I fill up the house with good food, and on the other hand, I get angry with her for eating. And she absorbs everything, sees everything. Sees me.

Sometimes I worry that she might grow up to be anorexic, but even more so, I worry that she will grow up to be fat. I won't be able to bear it if she grows up to be fat.

How will I be able to wake up from my hibernation and touch myself there a little?

Do something good for myself.

September 25, 2000

I anxiously awaited your arrival.

I felt fear and curiosity mixed together. Did the process resonate with you, were you able to give in to it?

I wondered what you gained from our first session.

There is something in this first session that can affect the entire course of therapy, and sometimes even determine its fate. Indeed, trust in a therapeutic relationship is the outcome of a process, but it begins forming right at the first session.

You entered, Tamar, a little timid and perhaps slightly disappointed.

I tried to read your eyes.

I felt how the stress was tingling in the tips of my toes. I felt all my senses becoming alert.

And you surprised me, Tamar, as you spoke from a place I didn't expect.

"You know, it was strange," you said.

"I got home, excited. I have never been on a journey like this before, without a diet, without pills, needles. Only me with the blank pages. But what was even stranger was that I had never been invited on such a journey by the therapist. Before every dieting attempt, I'd dwell on it for months:

should I do it, should I not, what to do. I would throw long 'farewell parties' of feasting on food. Every meal was 'the last supper,' and so, from the moment I declared a diet, I would add two more kilograms. No problem. I'll lose them next week anyway. Starting next week, I won't be able to eat so many things that I like anyway. I would always make sure to postpone the diet to the first Sunday of the month. And all of a sudden this, with no preparation, no mental readiness. Someone else tells me, come.

"You realize how different this is. And I haven't even addressed the therapy itself, the treatment. Nor do I understand this journaling, these choices."

I was certain you would focus on the difficulty in journaling, in not eating wildly, in trying to practice restraint. But you were elsewhere.

You told me about your strange feeling of beginning a therapy that was not your initiative. A treatment that was supposedly forced upon you. After all, it was my idea to begin with. Yes, you were taken by it. It appealed to you and fascinated you, but it really didn't come from you. You said more than once that you had never started a weight loss regime that wasn't your initiative.

Although the choice was yours, you felt odd, ambivalent, and hesitant. You tested the boundaries. On the one hand, you kept an eating journal meticulously, but on the other, you felt no desire to control, judge or take responsibility for the food itself.

I felt resistance mixed in with self-will and indecision. Is it the fear of another failure, self-disappointment, or my possible disappointment of you?

Is it the urge for destruction before we even began?

I wondered what I was supposed to reflect back to you, and what you should take with you when you left the session. What message, what insight? How to make you see that despite it seeming like nothing happened to you over the week, a lot has happened in it.

From reading the written pages, I saw and felt that you, Tamar, were controlled by a fixed idea of the term "diet." I felt that you operated from false beliefs and an enormous fear of failure. In your perception, a person dieting abstains from many types of foods deemed forbidden. And if he eats them, game's over.

For example, if a person eats a hamburger, pizza, ice cream, he is eating high-calorie foods, and is in fact, "ruining" everything. You, too, Tamar, are influenced by this way of thinking whereby success is the ability to abstain completely from those high-calorie, delicious foods. Not touch, not taste even a bite. But, in reality, things are quite different.

This notion gave me strength. I realized there was stuff to work on, and most of all, who to work with. I felt there was room for a process, for setting a path as I saw it. And since most of the therapy had to do with changing perception, I explained to you that in my belief, there are no "allowed or forbidden" foods, as long as we choose the food by our own will, enjoyment, and true hunger. There is no fault in eating high-calorie food, because beyond physical satiety, there is significance in the satisfaction and pleasure derived from food, and it's important to allow that. If you abstain from certain foods and experience long-term deprivation from them, it may trigger binge eating.

I felt the session allowed for a mutual examination of "what's what."

You kept looking at me, checking my responses, my facial expressions. And I did the same thing with you. I kept my eyes on your face, your hands. Even if I didn't stare at you directly, I made sure to be attentive to every movement, blink, and message, whether hidden or visible.

I felt as if you were testing me to see how present I was. How strong and how convinced.

I don't know what went on in your head, but I was consistent and continued showing you what I saw in your eating journals. I believed that something of what I said would reach you. Soften you.

***

Why do I insist on writing as a therapeutic tool?

What is it about these written pages that I believe can make you learn, understand, feel?

From the content, the order and organization, the detail, and even the size and shape of the handwriting, I learn a great deal more about the patient than what is said in the session. The manner of eating, the choices, the mood and the feelings are expressed in the writing even unintentionally. In this way, I try to understand the patient's eating and reflect back what I see.

Through his journaling and the mirror I provide, the person begins to feel and understand himself.

Sometimes that is enough to create a change, and other times it is only the impetus for other processes.

Over the years, I have learned to recognize the value of journaling as a therapeutic tool, and just as I have undergone changes as a therapist, so did they.

The pages started out as large quarto pages lined as intricate tables. The patients filled out their eating details according to countless guiding questions such as, "What did I eat?" "How much?" "When?" "What triggered the eating?"

The pages were cumbersome and perhaps somewhat depressing. Over the years, they shrunk down to a friendly size, and the tables were eliminated. But they were still plain and rigid. Later still, the pages were accompanied by a picture of a lie-detector machine, which indicated that the person had to report "nothing but the truth."

When I look back at those pages today, I am horrified at the lack of trust toward my patients. As mentioned, the pages gradually changed and became colorful, forgiving, with less threatening messages, less judgmental and more accepting.

The following pages were prepared like a mirror that reflected a person's eating and behaviors around food, whereas, the current pages carry a message that allows for and accepts the existence of the id (the impulse, urges, desires, aggressions, sexuality) that stirs each and every one of us in great intensities.

In the dieting process, we try to fight our most primal impulses by suppressing them. I wanted to demonstrate that they, too, have the right to exist in our life, and perhaps it is impossible to totally block them, as diet rules stipulate. And I thought I would inquire, try to find out if and how much we can restrain ourselves, give up, abstain and suppress our desires? What is in these dark places that yearns to surge forth while we try to curb it? Maybe we can try to acknowledge the existence of these dark places rather than forcing them shut.

In the treatment, I try to act as a mirror. Not discuss, judge or preach.

Everything is done gently since it is all so fragile and delicate. The patient is entrusting in my hands hidden realms that he is sometimes unaware of himself.

And I? I study them carefully with respect and awe.

***

And you, Tamar;

I tried to reflect back to you what I saw in your pages, which you filled out meticulously all week. Indeed, I saw a lot of food, but you wrote it down, stripped it of its chaotic nature, because journaling, even if done in retrospect, doesn't allow you to escape and can prevent unrestrained eating.

And so, it did.

You ate:

- Sandwiches from light bread – two.
- Rice – a lot.
- Pasta with Alfredo and mushroom sauce – a lot.
- A whole fish, and while oven baked and not fried, it is still a whole fish, which is a pretty large portion.

- Bamba[16] – a large bag.
- You munched on Burekas[17] and one or two vegetarian patties at work.

While this wasn't a major decrease in quantities that would lead to weight loss, the very journaling prevented eating quantities that would cause more weight gain. By the simple act of writing, one could see that despite the doubts, you were there for your own sake. You dared to see and begin to know and acknowledge your eating.

For me, that was a lot.

And with that you left, Tamar.

And it seemed to me you left encouraged.

---

[16]A snack made of peanut-flavored corn puffs.
[17]Savory stuffed pastries.

Yom Kippur—October 3, 2000

We met three times already, and up until now, I couldn't bring myself to write again, although I often think about starting this treatment, which would surely be interesting—if I go for it.

I have never addressed myself this way before—through writing—and it's almost like a journal I never wrote.

In our last session, which was really short, I said that all I could do right now is come and write down what I eat, more or less.

Ayelet said that was a lot.

I said I wasn't yet able to bring myself to eat less. When we went over what I ate, Ayelet said there were days that were really okay or not bad. Other days could have been good days if I had eliminated a few unnecessary binges.

That is a totally different approach—a wonderful one—that respects me, the fat person.

It doesn't dictate what I should eat in advance. There is something very appropriate and allowing about it.

I'm not yet committed to losing weight, and Ayelet's interpretation seems reasonable to me. I will decide when to start watching my weight, after all, she invited me, and I agreed. Meaning, I didn't decide on the timing, and there is a power struggle of when I will give in.

When will I give in?

As if it's impossible for me to give up this size, as if that is me, stubborn, childish, with no need or ability to put limits, restraint, apply myself, keeping parts of me unintegrated. Not connecting the human, with the animalistic. Not connecting the knowledge with the cessation. Not connecting the word in my head with the body's muteness.

No connection.

No integration.

As though if I give in, I'll give up my selfhood, that animalistic, wild, unrestrained, fundamental, uninhibited id, shapeless, which I have kept to myself, buried deep down, protected within these layers of flab.

Losing it would be losing the self I've protected ever since I can remember experiencing fantastic physical sensations and fulfilling them through eating.

Because there it all seems normal and legitimate somehow.

Perhaps (this is the first time I've thought about it), all the physical sensations that stimulate the nerves, that remained muddled in my childhood, I have fulfilled through sensual desire, through the food. Maybe I can't, or won't, lose it because it's a little like committing suicide.

And what will be left of me without the properly hidden id?

And also, I'll show you by not giving up everything.

So primitive and childish.

But don't judge; forgive, be forgiving.

And there is the sabotage and the rebellion.

Meir always says I'm a rebel, and he knows what only angels know.

My Meir.[18]

It's true; I always sabotage, I never let myself follow through with things.

Enjoy my handiwork all the way.

Be a child of God.

Be nestled as I know how, abundant, experiencing joy and happiness. When something succeeds, to give myself credit for it, and own the fruits of my labor.

With Meir, it's doing what he suggests: breathe next to things instead of being sucked into them. Be in a less understanding place, simply be, and know that everything I encounter is my reflection, whether similar or opposite. Approach things from a place of opportunity, a lesson, and find the light within me. Be a vessel of the light. Because there is no meaning to light without a vessel and none to a vessel without the light.

And I—I give myself and practice all this, but I always spoil it, hit walls and then drop everything I learned with him. Sinking deeper and deeper, instead of fusing the tools I already have, which Meir taught me. Some are physical tools, like breathing, vibrating, turning inward, and not eating animals. But somehow, I always sabotage all these.

Meir calls me a rebel. I consistently adopt everything he teaches me, yet push it away at the same time.

---

[18]Meir–a spiritual teacher and therapist Tamar and her family have visited for sessions and workshops ever since she got sick.

Never following through, so as not to succeed too much.

It's like having cancer, and adopting a healthier, better lifestyle, but not following through on it.

It's maintaining the diabetes.

It's eating healthily all day and then stuffing yourself something harmful, even if I don't enjoy it.

It's investing in work, giving my all; and when I experience success with a child, or with a few children; or in general, when I lead successful processes at work, I always make sure not to be present at the moment of joyful accomplishment, the moment of fame.

It's being behind the camera for days when they film a movie about work. I prepare, organize, make sure the staff and the children are in it, keeping their privacy and dignity. But when the camera turns to face me, I can't deliver, not even a professional statement.

I don't give myself that credit.

A rebel cause; who can tell me to give up my sabotage?

The sabotage: to punish myself, spoil it for myself, especially with my dearest ones, Nadav and the kids; to want it to be wonderful, but in the meantime, cause conflict, anger, and tension.

Not following through, rebelling so I can keep to my corner.

Never fully recover.

That's why it took me years to complete my M.A. because I never allowed myself to enjoy the esteem. I don't know how to make my simple daily life good enough so I can enjoy it.

Actually, come to think of it, I am so ascetic with my own private activities that even going to the mall by myself sometimes, or sitting in a café or on the beach with a girlfriend when I'm the initiator is so rare.

I hardly let myself enjoy what is available; I don't know how to enjoy what I succeed in. "So much judgment exists in your flabby, fat body, Tamar." I even look at myself from the outside when I'm in bed, taking a mental picture of myself while I'm inside and feeling self-disdain while doing so. Locking up my frightening, whorish femininity inside this body, so that it wouldn't go wild and lose itself in any way.

But this you already know, Tamar.

That when you look good, you run wild, you are attractive, you are instinctive, sensual and adulterous, and you cannot be trusted.

Because you already know that when you look good, Tamar, everything attracts you and you attract everything.

You betray those who love you and give in to outside temptation, merely for the sake of another physical pleasure, a pastime. You destroy solid relationships and follow the darkness, which leaves you with nothing but the bitter taste of loneliness.

What were you looking for in those years when you looked good? What was it?

So you placed the flab as your superego—the gatekeeper.

This way, there were no tests, no failures, no need for integration within the personality, no need for maturity.

Why are you crying over this now? You've known that since childhood and adolescence—everything seduced you, and you wanted it all, immoral, immoral, immoral!

Else, what business does an eleven-year-old girl have with a sixteen-year-old guy?

And how, in the army, you would flirt with the boyfriends of your close girlfriends, who loved you?

And enter into relationships with married officers, whose wives you knew; that always ended badly. So here are the morals—the gatekeeper—grabbing you by the throat so you won't go wild, covering you with a white, flabby layer, making you manly, so you are never an object of desire.

Because they pat me on the back, even men.

Because I'm huge and solid. Why would they hug me gently? That's ridiculous.

But how did I get carried away into all this? Because you only need to push a button.

Everything is filed in a dark, suppressed memory.

Everything there is tangled and scary.

Ayelet, Ayelet, what happened here?

It's not fair to arrive with such a load; it's heavy. But all that is not important. The treatment—here I gather myself, shaking it off and going back to the treatment. Because what is the source and what is inside is not operative.

We seek God in daily life, every day and every moment, in everything, find the meaning, the light. Not wait for special occasions. To all find how I benefit myself in all my actions, how I flow and nestle in the hammock of life.

And, in day to day, I'm all about eating, a little girl, knowing everything and yet knowing nothing. It helps me so much to

understand, as you said, Ayelet, that I see things in opposition.
All or nothing. Black or white. Primitive. What a pain.
What a pain to see things like that, to live like that.

Dieting is scary; you have to give up everything and do
everything differently, give up my lifestyle, it's an impossible
mission. And now, you come along and say, on the contrary.
Within what you are used to eating, just take off this, and
this, and you will lose. A little. How easy, unthreatening and
non-mission like.

This is daily life, with its ups and downs, and I so need you
to tell me "this pastry is unnecessary." I know that, but I'm a
kid, a baby, I need to hear it over and over again. I guess I am
impaired in this area and never really dealt with it.

Just like my center of hunger is impaired, so am I.
It's never hunger that has driven me to eat and not the
satiety that stopped me from eating. I think the hunger center
in my brain is deleted.

So is the field you pick your food from. When there
is food around, for me, it's like a blurry field. I pick from
indiscriminately—with no precedence—what is prettier, what
is tastier, what do I like more.

I eat everything and a lot of it.
How many types of food can I say I don't like?
But how come in all other areas, I have likes or dislikes, I'm
selective, I can choose, I'm refined, critical.
I need a hand. One that will guide me step by step and help
me give up that know-it-all theory place, the yes and no, and
the should and shouldn't.

It's all in my head, but I really need someone to guide me from the inside, through experience, through myself, to engage in a new dialogue with myself, that apparently, every non-fat person engages in before they eat.

It's like a though discipline that doesn't even exist in me. I have to practice creating such a discipline. It's like a skill I don't have at all and maybe never did, because up until now, it's always been either dieting—which means engaging in an imposed, temporary, tormenting and punitive suffering—or in mindless compulsive eating out of habit. My habits suck, and who cares where they come from. If I manage to treat them, what will blow up then?

Give yourself a chance to recover, Tamar. It's more than just recovering from obesity; it's recovering from the deepest wounds of the abysmal sadness inside you.

A sadness slowly shaped through my childhood, weaved in thin strands that grow and envelope my excessive being. There is always a squashed part inside that is best left dormant, sedated.

Please, don't wake up.

Let go of the pain, be a child of God, of simplicity and joy. Peel off the weightiness, the load.

Fly.

You're crying again.

And you're already forty.

Forty dimensions have lived through you. Gift it to yourself. You are good. What kind of snag has made you so bundled, smoldered, contracted? Look what an amazing surrounding you have, one that can take care of this little girl and guide her toward being a non-fat woman.

Everything is laid out for you. Supportive, loving and caring parents.

Nadav, pure goodness. Loves me, accepts me with all my ups and downs. With all this size. So stable. Never stormy. Always calm. And makes do with so little in our relationship. It's so easy to please him. It's so effortless.

What else do you need?

Just hold onto this. To him and to your kids.

Hold onto this world and all the good it can offer you.

Let go of the demons haunting you.

October 4, 2000

It was a "long" week, almost ten days. It could have easily turned into a disastrous one.

It was a holiday week, which is another substantial reason why it could be hard. Because any deviation from the routine can cause chaos. I knew it would be hard for you, Tamar, because you had just started your journey, and already had to tackle many potholes such as festive meals, rich with delicatessens; family gatherings; and lots of free time, without the boundaries of work. And you, as I suspected, easily went down the slippery slope of chaos.

But only a little.

Because there were pages, which, despite the difficulty, you filled steadfastly, and they guarded you against sinking completely.

You know, Tamar, when a person documents his eating on a daily basis, he really doesn't "get lost," neither to me as the therapist nor to himself. And perhaps, so I thought, you would not lose yourself—and we know how good you are at that.

The idea behind writing the eating journal is that you write the food sheet, the plan, the rules—which you are so used to getting from your caretaker—by yourself, without any external anchor to rely on. You plan for yourself. You are responsible for yourself.

This way, I believe we can try to break down your conscious and unconscious "anger" toward the "diet" or toward me as the therapist, who is supposedly in power.

I thought that, perhaps this way, we could prevent the struggle between you and the "impossible" diet and focus on your internal coping. I hope the journaling will give you an accurate mirroring of yourself so that you may become aware of your eating patterns and understand who controls them.

Ask yourself what you really want to eat, and why? And make your choice from this. Perhaps then, you could even enjoy the eating.

"Does it sound strange to you?" I asked.

"Yes and no," you answered.

"I understand that you can't 'suffer' for too long, or you can't eat according to a written plan for more than a few days, but I don't know any other way. Logically, I understand what you're telling me, but it's hard for me after so many years of sticking to diet plans, to think that any other way is possible. You see, Ayelet, for years I've gotten used to people telling me what to eat, how much and when. You realize that for years now when I was on a diet, I was not allowed to eat so many foods I like: cakes, chocolate, nuts, bread, cereal, yellow cheese, and so much more. I'm so used to suffering on a diet, to walking around hungry. And you talk to me about enjoying food? Do you understand the absurdity of this, to be able to enjoy it and lose weight? How will I lose weight if I eat all the things I like?"

"You're right," I replied, "I don't think that you can lose weight if you continue to eat everything in large quantities. But what I'm trying to tell you is that it's not about eating or not, you can eat some tasty, 'rich' food and some 'cheap' food (calorie-wise.) So, you can enjoy both worlds, and you get to choose how much, where and when.

"It reminds me that we once distinguished casual wear from Shabbat or holiday attire. Whereas today, everything is mixed up. What is the difference between regular days and holidays? We always dress up fancy. All the time. And the same goes for food. We eat rich, unique foods not only on special occasions but every day. So why wonder when everything gets jumbled, and rich, unique food becomes a daily routine?

"Perhaps this is where part of the change I am discussing lies?

"Perhaps if we could eat 'regular food' on 'regular days' and only eat festive foods on special occasions, we would actually be putting up boundaries that would help us even a little?

"During this festive holiday period, you slipped into those thought patterns where you told yourself, 'Oh well, I already messed up my eating, so let's mess up today and be more careful tomorrow.' But, to your credit, I must say that this time, everything was more moderate, aware and controlled.

"I remember you telling me how you cooked lunch, and it was usual for you and Nadav to go into the kitchen, each one contributing his share to the creation. Yes, with you is truly a creation infused with thought and imagination.

"You will also never say, 'I ate a salad,' just a salad. The salad will always be enhanced and delicately seasoned with raspberry vinegar, garnished with pomegranate seeds, served fresh in a hand-made clay bowl. Or, for instance, if you ate wheat berries, you wouldn't serve it like sticky rice, but puffed, each berry separate and cooked to perfection, with the proper texture and sprinkled with raisins and cinnamon.

"The way in which you describe what you prepared and ate feels like a pampering message.

"And when you are seized by an irrepressible binge, it seems that you no longer pay attention to the style and quality of the food. You eat for the sake of eating, so it doesn't really matter what the food looks like or its quantity.

"The main thing is the quantity.

"Pitas, spreads, quiches, oily filo dough pastries, crème cakes, and other cakes, what does it matter, when you have already 'forgotten' about the sugar that is flooding your blood. Luckily, you managed to give up the wine...but how is it possible to throw such a feast and completely abstain from the desire and pleasure involved in eating?

"Especially as the mega binge does not only arise from uncontrollable desire for food. With you, it has additional meanings, such as detachment, filling the void, or simply searching for warmth and some coddling.

"So how can we substitute one deprivation for another and expect to see a change we can stick with?"

"Many times the eating problem emerges in order to make it easier to cope with difficulties we cannot access, feel or solve. By temporarily 'numbing' and silencing these difficulties, we divert them from our path.

"With a conventional diet, we create a new frustration for ourselves, an alternate frustration that eventually often triggers increased eating.

"How long can a person surrender, sacrifice and suffer? He will eventually find himself needing some form of compensation for the deprivation he brought upon himself. And the deprivation is satisfied by the most basic, instinctual, and perhaps, somewhat primitive urge—by food.

"And the food, once consumed, causes weight gain.

"And we attempt to solve this weight gain by creating a new problem once again.

"We try to cope with our eating problem by finding no less difficult paths than those problems our eating was 'born' to numb, so as to hide it from ourselves.

"And the food, once consumed, generates feelings of guilt that send us looking for compensation once more, which leads to eating that produces a vicious cycle that repeats itself.

"And you, Tamar, so experienced with these places, as you have been there so many times. You would diet, lose 15 Kgs. (33 Lbs.), and gain them back with a surplus. And then, wear out and be left depleted of energy with a new top weight. How long can you restrict yourself and live in an ongoing genuine deprivation? So you abstain for a month or two, three at best and then…

"The longest time frame you were able to maintain a process of awareness was about a year. And you really felt good about yourself. You would walk three times a week and attend the support group you belonged to religiously. But even that attempt, like the previous ones, came to an end. And you have been in this vicious cycle for nearly fifteen years.

"I hope that through this treatment, we will try to facilitate eating from a choosing, accepting place for you.

"We will try to make the pleasure of eating legitimate; to restore your self-confidence in your decisions; and to reach a place where you will not be constantly governed by feelings of guilt.

"Your eating is driven by different sources. Discovering and identifying them may ensure your ability to cope and control them."

People who start a diet or treatment against binges have a tendency to make sweeping announcements such as 'Off limits!' 'I'm on a diet!' 'This is not on my food plan!' 'I'm going to focus on it and make it big time!'"

But the nature of these announcements is to dissolve.

Their magnitude makes them threatening and oppressive.

Announcements of this nature invite everyone into our plate, and our commitment becomes an obligation to everyone around us rather than a commitment to ourselves.

Many people allow themselves to cross the line and invade a fat person's privacy. They interfere with managing his body, needs, and desires while ignoring his right to privacy.

Such is the case with one of my patients, Hila, who is busy defining her own boundaries and just how deep she allows others to penetrate them.

In the following lines, I shall bring excerpts from her journal, where she talks about the pain, anguish, and mostly the disappointment with the closest people to her, who judge, criticize, and mainly invade her privacy.

Dad started up again today. "So, look in the mirror and see how much you eat." — "How can you eat after yesterday's restaurant?" (That was Mom.) What kind of a ridiculous question is that? Yesterday was yesterday and today is today, and that's it.

It's eight-thirty, and they're in my plate again. Oh, if I were only alone...

Ugh!

I feel like I have to please everyone all the time.

They tell me what to wear, check my plate, tell me who to be with.

And they're never really pleased with anything.

I'm getting fat, and I don't look like how they want me to look.

"And worst of all, she doesn't have a boyfriend."

And even if I have a relationship with someone, it's doomed already.

Galit is one of the few that gives me the strength to continue and believe and love myself.

I spoke to her a lot about the diet and how my parents simply don't accept the fact that I'm fat. Sometimes, it sounds like I'm a drunkard, but it's something so innocent—to crave food.

Galit claims, rightfully, that it's more important to be aesthetic, clean and groomed, and my grades are high for all these.

I feel like I need to come out and say, "Okay, at this point in my life, I'm not willing to give up any piece of chocolate. I like it like that, and I like to eat." That's how it is for now, and maybe it will take a long time until I decide to go on a diet again. But until then, I'm fat. And that's all there is to it.

Look at the inside, I'm not just my weight; I'm made up of many more things, and if you don't have the eyes to look inside, to penetrate the thick layer of fat, then too bad for you. Give it up.

Every time my Dad sees me eat he says, "Eat something… what's happening to you?"

"How can you live like that?"

"How was the concert last night, did you have anything to wear?"

"You've gotten wider." He gestured with his hand.

"Don't you want to do something? You'll end up doing what Irit is doing now (bariatric surgery)."

That was too much…so I got up and went to my room, and then he said, "That's it? You're offended, so you go down to your room?"

I cried on the stairs.

I'm calling Galit now. Only she understands.

Meanwhile, call waiting…come on…answer already…I hung up.

Why today? I tried to put on the last two pairs of pants that still fit me, but alas.

They simply didn't close.

That's how the morning began, so I wore a skirt.

I prepared clothes for the following day on the chair: a brown, wrinkled skirt with a white shirt and a vest; I even prepared socks.

I know I gained a lot of weight.

I'm not willing to give up. It's simply two parallel lines that won't meet right now.

And I can only solve this problem by buying larger clothes.

Galit is the only one in the world who can understand.

And, Dad, you're a moron, stupid and insensitive.

Now he called to ask if I had the newspaper. What he wanted to ask is if I was okay. Why can't he just ask? Or was he really calling to ask if I had the newspaper? In which case, he's really insensitive.

I got a hold of Galit on the second time. She says my Dad is superficial, and she's right.

She has no idea how much.

She was so offended for me. What a superficial world. I suddenly feel like hugging Shaul (part-time lover) and telling him I love him and that he makes me feel pretty, the prettiest.

Amir loves me.

Merav loves me.

Anat loves me.

Meira loves me.

And Nava, of course.

Aside from them, I can't say that my being fat doesn't affect my other girlfriends.

And I love myself so much.

I think I'm strong.

I cried all right, but only a little.

And I went on crying, like I wrote a few pages back. That today I woke up knowing I would cry.

I wonder what will happen in the end. I think people will slowly realize that I'm fat, and no one will die from it. And if they do, it's their problem. I told Galit that my Dad doesn't know me.

Our Self is our Private Temple

Treating the world behind the food is a long and Sisyphean process.

It involves chronic repetitiveness that drains and wears out both the patient and the therapist. The success of such a treatment is not only measured by how many kilograms the person has managed to drop and does not culminate in a numeric figure on a scale. This success means arriving at a new place—a place where the person feels good about himself and his body on a physical and emotional level. And this place is individual for every person.

And, Tamar, I would like you to try to view this path as an ongoing one, with bends and curves. Success is sometimes the mere ability to walk, to keep walking.

I will try not to make you weary, but I would like to say a few words about one of the main traps along the way. This supernatural thinking controls many people's eating behaviors.

Some people are controlled by irrational thoughts and beliefs that magnify their problems in relation to food, in relation to their perception of themselves and in relation to their eating behaviors.

For instance:

"If the day started on the wrong foot, and I ate a croissant, then it's a lost day, and it doesn't matter how much and what I eat."

"I have an event in two days, and I won't be able to lose my excess weight by then anyway, so nothing matters anymore."

"I have so much weight to lose. Why bother starting?"

"I'll never be what I want to be."

Tamar, it seems to me that you think similarly quite often. Once you have started to binge, you won't try to stop it or offset it later. You get into the mode of "all hell breaks loose" and eat whatever is available, indiscriminately.

Or if you were careful all day and slipped a little at night, eating something you feel wasn't planned, the entire day is doomed and can be destroyed because it is not as perfect as you thought it should have been. And so, no day can be completely "clean," and you continue the repetitive cycle of fasting-binging that doesn't lead you to any true change.

So where are you, Tamar?

Don't run away from yourself.

Don't run away from me.

Just be.

***

"It was different," you said.

I didn't feel the stress involved in dieting, but I also didn't feel the excitement and waves of joy that fill me every time I succeed in starting a weight loss program. I was very relaxed and tried to do what you said. Just writing down. Thinking and writing down. Not that I was thrilled by what I saw, but I wrote it."

"I understand a little of what you're going through," I said, "because there is no solid plan or strict and clear framework. In all that 'isn't,' you must find what there 'is.' And it's hard, scary."

I did feel the dilemmas emerge right at the beginning of the journey. And the resistance threatened to break the rules before they were even laid.

And you came, abundant and real, somewhat present and somewhat not.

Yes, despite it all, you came.

And you wrote—everything.

Detailed, organized. What you ate, when, how much. You managed to document your eating in a true fashion. You wrote the light bread sandwiches Nadav makes for you each morning, the aromatic fresh pastries that the pastry shop in your workplace produces every day. You described in detail the delicious food you make at home. The soy dishes, the high-calorie pasta, the fresh fish you bake in lemon and herbs, and the delicious bread Nadav bakes in your bread maker. You wrote it all, even if it was a lot.

And it was a lot.

In quantity, in variety and mainly in frequency. All the time, nearly every hour.

The mere journaling had a lot in it for me. Readiness, self-attentiveness, cooperation.

"Is that a diet?" you asked, "I didn't even feel myself making an effort like I'm completely committed. I didn't walk around hungry, I didn't suffer, and besides journaling, I didn't do anything."

I felt that you were disappointed and perhaps even mad—at yourself? At me?

Disappointed by the fact that, despite your decision, nothing happened. That despite your effort, you were unable to give up and eat only "diet" things, that if you took a project upon yourself, how come you are not really running it as one?

And I listened, smiled. That's how you begin.

I loved the uncertainties, the way of thinking that reflects the difficulty in creating a change in the eating patterns.

And what was on those pages that disappointed you so, Tamar? That drew a failure for you?

And you asked, "How can I eat normal food and lose weight? You noticed I ate all the food in the house. I didn't cook especially for myself, I didn't buy myself low-calorie groceries, I ate normally. Yes, I tried to think, plan, but ultimately I ate as usual."

Sure enough, there was real, delicious, pleasurable food there; "forbidden" food, "non-diet" food, homey food: meatballs in tomato sauce, festive fish dishes, sweet Challah bread, Matzo Ball soup, homemade honey cake.

And I said;

"Success is not just about what we eat, but when and how much. Success lies in the emotion, thought, awareness and insight involved in eating."

Journaling, coming to sessions, coping with disappointment—that is success.

"I have no doubt that the very fact that you wrote what you ate led to mindful eating, even if you weren't aware of it. No drastic changes, yet you no doubt ate less, even if you didn't notice it.

"You lost 1.7 Kgs. (3.74 Lbs.) That's a fact."

October 7, 2000

Do I really want to lose weight?

Or have I stumbled upon this adventure by chance?

Meir says there is no such thing as chance. I agree with him. There is some order to creation, and as part of this order, in regard to my obesity, it seems my time has arrived.

But for real or like always?

Why should I lose weight?

Because I'm afraid to die. Is that a good enough reason?

And maybe one should desire to live instead of being afraid to die.

And maybe I get a little suicidal with this fat all the time, playing dangerous games with life.

I love the twilight zone of danger.

Once, during a time when I looked good when I wasn't so heavy, I would race with guys when standing with my motorcycle at a red light.

If a handsome guy would stand next to me, I'd lure him into a race.

It could have ended badly on numerous occasions.

At the beach, too.

At times when I would return from the army, I would stop at the beach in winter before heading home. I would plunge deep into the waves, even when it was very stormy, swim farther, waiting for the waves to take me. Teasing them. I would return to the shore breathless, choked, coughing and puking seawater.

In Nomad and Viper *by Amos Oz,[19] when the viper bites the heroine, she drops to the side of the path. I have always wanted to replace her, in that sweet surrender into the alluring arms of death.*

But in the end, I always want to come back.
You're such a coward.

How do you really feel the desire to live?
Do I fill myself with food to feel alive or dead?

---

[19] Amos Oz is an Israeli writer, novelist, journalist, and intellectual, as well as Israel's most famous living author.

October 10, 2000

I was convinced you were on the fence, watching from the sidelines, testing boundaries.

I was surprised; you're in the game, involved.

Granted, you still don't give up the large food quantities; you still eat, and a lot. But you also understand that showing up, journaling, and thinking are part of the process. And it's not only measured by your ability to eat 1,500 calories a day. Up until now, you have never been involved in treatment— you were always on a mission, and to succeed on a mission, you must enlist yourself. You must be totally in it. Yet, most of the problem lies in that totality.

While your achievements have yet to be reflected in a significant weight loss, they are reflected in your way of thinking, relating, and understanding that a menu or a structured food plan are not the right working method for you.

Tamar, you still have a lot of food—rich, colorful and diverse—just like you.

There is still no behavioral change, aside from detailed, ordered journaling.

There is no major calorie reduction, and therefore, there is no significant weight loss.

It was clear to me that if I weighed you in this meeting, the scale would show a weight gain. I debated with myself quite a bit. In my approach, the weight is not a goal, but a means. The goal is to try to disconnect the patient's feelings, his view of himself, and his behaviors from the number on the scale.

It is very important for me, Tamar, that you feel yourself part of the experience, not just as dependent on an absolute scale devoid of any feeling. Weight is merely a numeric figure, and as such, has no feelings, no thoughts, and no ability to assess behaviors. It's a cold, factual measure that discloses information about caloric balance.

A number cannot be the objective of treatment.

I believe that it is wiser to speak of the place we aspire to reach. Such a place is made up of your own experience with your body, with yourself, and with the emotional state you are in. And the place? It can change.

It's subjective; it's not dictated by weight charts of any kind. It is yours only, and you can find it and settle in it.

A review of the professional literature in the field shows that the best way to determine how much a person should weigh should include:

A cessation of limiting diets.

Attempts to cope with eating binges and controlling them.

Enjoyable physical exercise.

Allowing each and every person to find their Set Point throughout the course of treatment.

Most patients have a hard time accepting such an approach since it sometimes entails giving up the possibility of reaching a goal weight that lives up to their fantasies. The ability to give up becomes especially hard in light of the diet industry that enhances and amplifies the fantasy of ideal weight. The industry gives off an impression that every person can supposedly choose his goal weight by simply picking the suitable diet to bring him to that goal, and the rest will take care of itself. But the facts are discouraging and speak for themselves—it doesn't work.

Thus, one should:

1. Avoid choosing an absolute goal weight and focus on developing eating habits, awareness, and ability to cope with binges (if there are any.)
2. It is important to understand that weight fluctuates depending on the fluid balance in the body. Therefore, weight does not always reflect the body's objective state accurately.
3. In assessing a person's goal weight, it's important to refer to the weight and personal and family history.
4. A proper assessment of a healthy body weight should be approximately 10 percent under the highest weight of that person before he began treatment.[20]

I shared with you information that may be a bit frustrating.

---

[20]Garner, David M. Paul E. Garfinkel, Ed. *Handbook of Treatment for Eating Disorders*. Second edition, The Guilford Press, NY, 1997.

I was worried you might say, "Fine, then I don't even want to make an effort. I can't be thin anyway." But you were silent.

And I said, "I believe it's not easy for you to listen to what I'm saying. But even losing 20 Kgs. is considered a change. A healthy change for sure. And perhaps, Tamar, that is a good thing, since it's hard to think about losing 45 Kgs. anyway. In any case, our use of the scale must also be controlled; we should use it only when you feel it benefits you."

I felt like you understood; you didn't feel upset. But I still thought it would not be right to weigh you, Tamar. Because if you saw a weight gain on the scale, it could ruin the small, rickety bridge between us. Whereas if you saw a weight loss, you would be positively reinforced for behavior that shouldn't otherwise be rewarded. So, that message may have been confusing and perhaps even hindering.

What is important for me is to make sure that although you are still hesitant, and not fully in the process, and though there isn't significant weight loss yet, you will continue. Right now, I believe that we must simply stick to the treatment and move forward.

And you?

You looked at me, smiling. I felt a sigh of relief.

"You know, Ayelet," you said, "I rather like it. I feel that letting go of the weight gives me a certain comfort. You allow me to feel that I'm not only measured by how much I weigh, but also by what I have done, how I felt, how I behaved. It's certainly liberating.

"You know how anxious I am before every weighing. You know how much the weight tips me off. It determines how I feel, it can even dictate my entire day.

"And now you're taking it off the pedestal. Removing its sting. It feels nice. Yes, it's a little confusing, because how will I know if I was good or not? I'm so used to it knowing and deciding for me. But even so, I like the idea. Though there will be times when it will be important for me to be weighed, and I won't always feel comfortable with the uncertainty. But right now, it really suits me. And I'm not afraid of not being able to handle what the scale says."

And you left with your head held high.

In Anat's case, I also tried to bring her to view the scale as a powerless object and understand that she is the one granting it the power and the key role it plays in her life.

I tried to help her look at it from a slightly different perspective so that she could strip away its power and how it affects her feelings and self-esteem.

Anat has been coming to my clinic for years, as I watch her shrivel, wilt.

She seems to be moving, but it's more like crawling.

She seems alive, but not for real.

Something in her is extinguished.

Something is hardly breathing.

Anat, thirty-five, pleasant looking. An economist. Married with two children. Household, workload—and weight. Routine. Exhausting. Draining.

Over the years, Anat gained more and more weight as if she could not get enough. The more weight she gained, the more her husband criticized her. Every time he put his foot down and announced, "Either I walk away, or you lose weight!" she would get panic stricken, pull herself together, work hard, and lose weight.

Five or six kilograms later, she would desert the battlefield, defeated, settling back into heaviness, lethargic and lifeless. Until next time. She would become proactive only for him. She had long since lost interest in herself. But can someone help themselves only to please another person? Tears flood her eyes frequently.

It is hard for her to find the power within herself, to understand and to know what she wants, what could stimulate her, breathe some life into her. Sometimes, it seems as if she yearns for nothing.

She simply gets by.

In addition to her fatigue, her body refuses to cooperate with her, causing her great frustration. For once she enlists herself and succeeds in watching her food, give up and reduce quantities, she is never adequately rewarded. She doesn't receive positive reinforcement, not from the scale, which refuses to respond fast enough, and certainly not from her husband, who wants tangible results and for tens of kilograms to simply disappear.

And she is so far from that.

Which causes an immediate relapse. For how do you reconcile the logical understanding that this is a slow process that requires perseverance to succeed, and the feeling that nothing is important and that you will never feel good about yourself?

And then, the relapse is fast and brutal.

She eats limitlessly, knowingly, yet consuming carbs and sugars, rice, hi-calorie sandwiches, snack bags, nuts, almonds—thousands of calories.

And she has no power in her to stop, to get a grip. She feels the weightiness of her body, sinking into a caressing lull of lost senses. For that is what the food does best—numb the feelings, the pain, the disappointment.

And then, she is overcome by guilt and self-contempt. Completely crushed, drenched in a sea of calories that wreaks havoc on her body. And on and on again.

How can something such as a scale, a lifeless piece of iron, devoid of insight and feeling, bring failure and destruction? How can a scale build and destroy worlds all at once?

What is it all about?'

What is it about its supernatural power that makes people observe it and deem it such an undisputed authority?

A boring, plain device.

Yet this boring device seals fates. It tells us how to feel about ourselves and about our bodies, whether we look good, feel good.

Whether we behaved properly or deviated, bluffed.

It can bring us much joy and at the same time drag us to the pits of despair.

Yet these are only numbers on an iron scale.

Anat and I decided that she should stop being weighed. We would no longer allow the scale to run and dictate her life. We would not let it decide for her what kind of a person she is, how she behaves, what she does, and whether she is of value or not.

It wasn't easy, because Anat never really fought with it, never tried to argue with it or question its verdict. She would weigh herself and cry, weigh herself and beat herself up. The same is with her husband. They both have her in a panic, paralyzed. She tries to please them and fails. She tries to satisfy their desires and fails every time anew.

But, whereas with the scale it happens without words, her husband says a lot of hurtful, piercing words.

"Look at yourself."

"I'm embarrassed to be seen in public with you."

"Everyone has elegant, aesthetic, thin wives, and you?"

"Can't you shut your mouth a little? I don't understand what the problem is, why can everyone else do it and you can't?"

Maybe because these aren't her needs and wishes. Those that are, she dares not feel, recognize, or wish for herself.

And then, she crashes.

Letting go of the scale wasn't easy.

Did the difficulty stem from the fear that there would be no more external factor to be blamed, mad at or fought with?

Or perhaps the problem is deeper and scarier.

From now on, Anat should only rely on herself. Only she can give herself reinforcement, only she can give herself "grades," only she can tell herself what happened, how she behaved, how she feels about her body and what her self-worth is.

No more external judges or external orders dictating to her.

She is on her own.

And that is scary.

She was frightened; she had been bound to the scale for years. She was used to weighing herself every day, sometimes even a few times a day. She was used to punishing herself with it, by endlessly beating herself:

"Look how worthless I am."

"Ugh, I ate 200 gr. of pistachio again."

"Look how I can't restrain myself, as soon as everyone is asleep, I sit down in front of the TV with a pack of cookies or a bag of M&M's."

"It doesn't matter how careful I am, I'll never be thin, never be worthy, never look good."

She often uses the scale to express self-anger, cry because of it, eat because of it. What will be without it?

She looked at me. Her eyes glistened.
She glanced at it.
Lowering her head.

And I don't know where this will take us.

I don't know how much strength she will have to fight for herself.

But I would like to believe that this step will awaken dormant powers in her. I know she can find them in herself and enlist them to her benefit.

I looked at her again.

I want it for her.

I hope she does too.

Two years later.

Anat is still stuck.

Still finding it hard to break the cycles of food that run her life so powerfully.

The attempts to let go of the scale have also failed, and she finds herself sinking down to her neck, slowly wallowing within herself, heavy.

October 25, 2000

"That's it, this time, I hope it's a true beginning, and that the process of weight loss will begin."

Each time, I try to generate optimism, in me, in you. Blow wind into the sails that are gazing down. Just like now.

I try to be practical and spoke about situations that trigger eating.

Many times, we create the situations for eating, seemingly without noticing, but really, they are an alibi for our hidden desires to eat. And, perhaps if we would be more mindful, we would succeed in refraining from certain situations that we know would trap us into eating.

For example, we stuff our pantry or fridge at home with different pastries, snacks, new ice cream flavors, and expect ourselves to know they are around, yet to abstain from eating them. This is hard and sometimes impossible. Or we create situations that invite eating and drag us into uncontrollable binges.

Tamar, how many times do I hear about a social dinner you organized and the massive quantities of food that you laid on your plate? You are unable to give up anything. You try out, check, excited by every discovery of a new delicacy.

Sometimes, you go back for a second helping, another side dish, desert, salad.

And by that time, the quantities are truly out of hand, and you are no longer mindful of your eating because what does it matter if you eat 2,000 or 3,000 calories?

Often times, the eating event could have been prevented if we were able to think beforehand and try to understand what we truly want, need and feel at that specific moment. Is it really hunger? And if it is hunger, is it a real physical one or an emotional one?

Sometimes we think we are hungry, but these feelings are really a signal to other needs we have, which we find hard to fill or touch on, such as love, physical contact, warmth. In which case, the food in its most materialistic level cannot help, because the real hunger is not for food.

And it happens a lot with you.

And you, Tamar?

Every night, when all the family members are asleep, you lie on the couch in the TV room, staring at the flickering images, not always attentive, and snacking. On whatever there is. This is your therapy hour.

Alone with the food. No one watching, no one asking.

Neither do you.

And you eat, mindlessly, slices of light bread with spreads, leftover savory snacks, and sometimes, you are not too lazy to heat up the leftovers from dinner.

Lying around.

You and the food.

Many times, I hear you say that what triggers you is the smell of food or the very knowledge that lunch is being cooked or pasties are being baked in the next room. And then, it doesn't even matter if you're hungry or not, if it's tasty, or whether you want it. You eat because it's there, and it arouses all your senses and desires, so like a junkie, you don't think, don't know, and eat.

I examined you closely, Tamar. Your size, your aesthetics.

I find myself thinking that if you only managed to lose about 20 percent of your weight. What would change? How would you look? What would be revealed under these immense fat deposits?

It's not just fat. It's layers of restrained sexuality, a wild id that is bubbling inside you, yearning to break free. Aggression refined by cynical humor and maybe righteous pretense or a woman who runs a normal life in a warm household, a steady job, friends. Yet under the surface, urges are stirring, which you consciously or unconsciously choose to repress.

This behavior enables you to live in the sophisticated super-ego realms you have developed throughout your life.

And how do they come into play?

In the jokes you crack all the time and in your manner of speech, which feels like you're performing an ongoing standup comedy. You are the main character as well as the secondary characters, the set designer and lighting designer. Everything is colorful, juicy and even seductive to some extent.

In my wildest fantasy, I would say that if you lost weight and regained your appealing size, that is, become good-looking, attractive, wild, you would drown in a sea of lust, tasting all the wonders of the Garden of Eden, which you have prevented access to by building those walls of silence around your body.

You would go out with countless men, experience wild and maybe even perverse sex, seek experiences that push you to the edge, that raise your level of excitement to the top.

And I saw all that size shrink and soften. The sinking belly disappeared, the little buttocks winking mischievously and the slender legs inside the stockings. The double chin dissolving and your face smiling in relief. I saw the mini-skirts and the dolled up platform shoes, the tight shirts and the pants without elastic bands.

And mostly—I imagined you, different.

And I wanted it.

For you.

Like an onion, every layer peeled off brings tears.

It's one thing to peel off, but to remain naked?

With no protection?

That is far more complicated.

Nudity invites closeness and intimacy; deeper, penetrating, threatening.

Nudity symbolizes a release from chains that you may have bound yourself in over the years.

And I ask myself, what is right for you, and is it possible that it's not right for you to lose weight?

Tamar, I don't know how much you can create this significant change in the present stage of your life. For many people, being thin is scary, and they have a hard time experiencing themselves as thin even though it is such a yearned for place in their fantasy.

There are many myths around thinness that are hard to cope with and can be frightening.

1. Thin women are perceived as cold, unaffectionate, self-centered.
2. They are expected to be successful, perfect, which takes away the alibi for failure. "It's okay not to succeed if you're fat, but if you're thin, what's your excuse?"
3. Thin women are considered more attractive and sexier. But not every woman can contain the feelings of being a sexual object, and it may arouse anxiety in her as well as a fear of being taken advantage of. Some women have a hard time handling their sexual desires, putting boundaries on them, and since thinness is perceived as projecting more sexuality, it can be threatening.
4. Thinness is perceived as creating an illusion of power and fewer boundaries, which arouses panic of an overpowering, "external invasion."
5. Thinness may cause fear of other women who perceive them as competition.
6. Thinness suggests giving up weakness, pain, and sadness, which no one will notice about thin women and their needs.

And where do I see these in you, Tamar?

First, in the sexuality, which we have briefly touched on. You present yourself as full of desires and urges, you talk about a past full of sexual promiscuity, longingly recalling how you were an attractive, good-looking, sexy woman and your love for unrestrained debauchery that characterized your youth. Would I be wrong if I said that the obesity, in part, is meant to keep you from these lustful eruptions that could easily ruin your marriage and family life? It is no coincidence that you gained weight after giving birth to your eldest daughter. Perhaps you were afraid that if you continued to feel attractive and sexy, nothing would stop you from the boisterousness of expressing your sexuality. When you're fat, very fat, it's hard to feel your sexuality, or that you are pretty and attractive, in which case, there is something stronger than us that protects us from ourselves and from our burning desires.

There are other things that scare you about being thin. I believe it has to do with your relationship to women. The fact that you are a fat woman places you in an unthreatening position compared to other women. You have a lot of power in you, Tamar, some of which is intimidating. Imagine you thin on top of all that?

There is something in the fat that softens your presence, enables unintimidating closeness and restrains some of that power.

You are a vibrant, interesting woman; a leader, one who takes charge, isn't afraid of conflict, a warrior; a woman of vision, goals, and many aspirations. And you have infused all these with passion and vitality, which makes you a fascinating, lively person. So imagine if you were slender, too?

I think that even when I met you for the first time, and one of your girlfriends told me about all the qualities you possess, said to myself, "Well, but she's so fat."

So then we talk about losing weight and your hopes to be elsewhere, and we realize that it would not be easy for you to be elsewhere either. Especially as you choose the extremes.

Everything about you is big, including the size. Ten excess kilograms aren't enough. Only a colossal overweight will block you and enable you to "enjoy" the indirect benefits it provides.

October 27, 2000

I think the last session was very powerful for me, Tamar. We sat opposite each other.

Close.

The first rain drops falling on my clinic window, the smell of freshness in the air.

We looked at each other. There was tension mixed in with excitement. The first session in which we decided to read to each other what we had written so far. Each one read aloud her feelings and thoughts. I thought this sharing would perhaps give you an added dimension on top of the usual sessions. I believed that if you read aloud what you had written until then, you could look at yourself from a different perspective. One of change. When a person is in the midst of undergoing therapy, it's hard for him to watch himself from the side and fathom the distance he has covered. I believed that if you watched yourself from the outside, you would feel things more intensely and maybe even deepen their presence in you.

And I chose reading because I thought that the experience of seeing the therapist's perspective could benefit you. If you understood my way of thinking, the essence of what guides me in my work, you would be able to deepen and internalize those insights and maybe even adopt some of them.

You spoke, and I listened.

I spoke, and you listened.

A lot.

For me, it was a genuine experience. It was interesting and exciting at the same time, involving vulnerability with insight, slight embarrassment, and relief. I stripped myself of the therapist's role. I expressed my fears, insecurity, vagueness, my desire to lead you to a better place, my strong wish for us to succeed in creating change and mainly my belief that it is possible. Whereas you, Tamar, spoke about yourself, about being stuck. About fifteen years of burdening fat. About the fear that this may be your last chance to try to lose weight. You don't believe in yourself that much anymore. You don't believe in your ability to be consistent in a framework, to account for yourself and to eat less. The ongoing attempts to drop weight have exhausted you.

You are heavy and tired.

I read you a poem I wrote.

> A chain of water wrapped around your drowning
> Body
> Choking constricted rings
> From the pits of your somber throat
> Tearing its chords
> Blackened with the rotting
> Of time

You nodded.

You pay a heavy price, you said, a dear and painful one—from a health standpoint as well as your inner feelings. Health-wise, you are plagued with illnesses, all of which are life-threatening. In terms of yourself, you may have learned to function in this size, but it takes a toll. You are always hot and sweating. On trips, you move heavily, and there are some sites you have to give up on reaching because you know you won't be able to walk them. Climbing the stairs is out of the question. Buying clothes that you really like, with a sexy flair, is something you have given up on a long time ago. You make due with wearing tents, and albeit nice ones, plus-size stores have a limited selection to begin with.

But above all, from the moment the fat took over your life, you have been forced to place yourself differently. In social situations, you joke about yourself and your excess fat, perhaps so that others won't.

A great deal of your sense of humor is geared toward examining yourself under the social magnifying glass. Because you're safer, protected that way.

It's not easy for you being this size, this different, yet you remain that way.

Tamar, I wonder if you can get in touch with your feelings without being overwhelmed by them. Can you live with such strong emotional and sexual needs without being swallowed by them? Or must you acknowledge the fact that in order to live in peace with yourself, you have to bury them deep and accept their loss?

What does that mean to you? Could it be your way of restraining yourself and abstaining from expressing sexuality? In which case, you may have nothing left but to unleash them through these eating binges full of lust and pleasure.

And maybe if these needs aren't blocked by the fat, they might have no boundaries. So, you place a boundary. A painful one, yet a boundary.

You nod in agreement.

You feel that my questions touch you in genuine places.

Your eating has a lot of passion in it. In the way you talk about food and in the sensual way you serve it. Binges are very similar to a wild sexual act. I recall one patient who would systematically go down to the nearby deli each night, buy five to six ice cream cones and "shove" them one after the other, and only then would she "calm down" and manage to fall asleep.

It is similar with you, only less organized, more erratic, whatever is in hand's reach. Snacks, leftover cake, fruit, everything you shouldn't have because of your sugar. Just like the "forbidden" sexual promiscuity.

You seemed to me a little upset. Not just by the inner revelation, but by the fact that you were able to bring up all the gushing intensities stirring inside you, talk about them, see them, and show them.

You were a little surprised by your ability to be fully present in the session.

You were terrified and said, "How did I manage to be so open and so allowing? I can't believe I opened myself up so easily, how quickly I let down my guard."

It scared you, and I was afraid that this openness could eventually block you. Perhaps there is something about these sessions that may cause you to say or do things you didn't plan in advance or didn't think you would do.

And then, you would regret it and run away.

But you can also look at this partial giving in as something good, calm, enabling, opening. I don't really know, but I feel that you were comfortable here, in a safe and protective environment.

And where was I?

Excited.

Curious to know what was going on with you beyond the things you told me. I was very curious about how you saw my role as your therapist. Do you experience the Ayelet in me that is hiding behind the therapist's role? Tamar, can you see the two Ayelets playing, deceiving? The Ayelet that peeks and quickly runs to hide. The Ayelet that touches you but doesn't allow herself to be touched. The Ayelet that sometimes wants so much, but is really so embarrassed and afraid.

Because a therapist is supposed to restrain his needs and desires and try to be as upright as possible. But, deep inside me, I needed you to discover a little of what I am trying to hide behind in my anonymous cloak. To learn about me without having to speak about myself. To sense my real character although it has no place or permission to step forth, by virtue of being a therapist.

It's interesting how preoccupied I am in my image as reflected in your eyes, how much I really want to be a solid container for you, an emotional and supportive entity that can help protect you from yourself, Tamar. Yet, I wanted so much for you to discover my other personality, which isn't satisfied by simply giving and wishes to receive without having to ask for it.

As always, you were present, massive and amazing.

That is what's so fascinating about you.

You hide inside this size. Vulnerable. Wanting to be caressed, to be revealed for the genuine, passionate, tender and little Tamar that you are.

Just like I want to but never say.

Size and fat often arouse a feeling in us that the person is repulsive, gross. Whereas I see in you gentleness, tenderness, and a rich spiritual world.

It is especially evident in your verbal ability, your picturesque writing and your emotionally exuding poems.

On my birthday, you chose to congratulate me:

Ayelet

Color, under thin paleness

Brown, volcano, under snow.

A large life within a small life

And nothing is as quiet as it seems.

I could see that under your strong, authoritative guise, you really wanted to allow yourself to come out.

To wallow in weakness, laziness, fatigue, vulnerability.

And indeed, through the process of writing, you felt the panic take over you.

You touched, and panicked.

It was too strong, too consuming, too invasive.

Many fantasies longing for adventure, for pleasure. Desires whose current presence was hard to come to terms with in your calculated, conservative lifestyle.

That was where the food came in to seemingly smooth over everything; to build protective walls on the one hand and to prevent access to you on the other. The fat was restraining and burdening. It put boundaries. It was painful, yet prevented the kind of coping that entails a different kind of pain.

And you were in the middle. Torn, uncertain. The price you were called to pay was too heavy to carry.

In illness, in weight, in sweating on hot summer days, in thinking that your children may be embarrassed by your appearance.

When did it all begin? When was the choice made?

Perhaps somewhere, years ago, when you were a little girl in kindergarten. Good and pleasing. A girl any mom would be proud of. But you were already paying the price for it. You ate under fear, distress, unfulfilled fantasies; to occupy space and presence, to disappear.

You gave up on yourself, your needs, especially in light of your dominant brother, who occupied the entire house and left no space for you. He was waited on, his needs were fulfilled, which at times left you to fend for yourself and fulfill your needs on your own. This was when food began to provide for you everything that you couldn't demand and receive. And so, you found yourself a niche that was all yours; pampering, nurturing, without having to wait for the rest of the family to become available and listen to what you truly needed and wanted.

There was no malice or negligence involved. It was a combination of a child who needed a lot of attention compared to a brother who demanded and received a lot more than you.

So, you found it on your own—in food.

Food became a place where you didn't give up. You controlled, managed, decided and mostly gave to yourself.

During adolescence, so you said, you were already big but sexy and attractive, not huge. You dared, experimented, from a young age, with "forbidden" pleasure. Everything big, with full senses on.

Mostly away from home—not at home.

There was something wild, captivating, and passionate.

At times I can see you in that light, vibrant, uninhibited.

And I?

I'm trying to go along with you on a therapeutic journey without patronizing. I won't try to change you, but try to impart to you different ways of thinking and behavior that will help you run your eating differently and handle chaos.

Tamar, I'm trying to steer you to finding out what you really want to eat, why, when and how much. So that you will learn to create your menu according to your likes, needs and the life situations you encounter on every given day.

For example, today I know you have an evening event that will include rich, delectable food. Try to figure out how to organize your day so that you will make it to the evening with enough calories to "spend," yet not too hungry, so that you don't lose control of your eating. And then, from a choosing perspective, you can examine the food being served and ask yourself, "What do I want to eat the most? What is 'worth it' for me? What will gratify and satisfy me?" And then, eat.

Satiety is a combination of fullness and pleasure. If one of these parameters is lacking, we're not really gratified by the eating and want more and more.

If we eat a giant salad, we may be full, but we will be lacking the element of pleasure that usually accompanies eating carbs. Or alternately, if we eat chocolate, we may enjoy it, but we won't be full.

So what do you think, Tamar? Can you enjoy eating without feeling guilty?

You were silent. In no hurry to respond.

Finally, you said, "I know there is an aspect to eating that I enjoy. Tasty, diverse food, partly fattening. I can enjoy that. It's usually the type of food I eat with friends and family. It's 'better' or more 'normal' food. I eat large quantities of it, but I think that if I were only to eat this type of food, I'd maybe be chubby—overweight by 10–12 Kgs. Average fat. The 'bad' eating is the other, 'sick' one.

"It's the one in which I put 'sad,' boring, fattening, jumbled, tasteless food into me. The kind I eat in addition to the 'happy' food, alone, at night, in front of the TV or during the day, offhandedly, just because it's there. Like a dry piece of bread that I happened to walk by or last night's cookie, all dried up on the kitchen counter. This food is dead food. Empty.

Devoid of happiness. I think that's the food that makes me so fat.

"And then, my guilty conscience slowly takes over. It grows and becomes a terrible monster that beats me mercilessly:

'How can you do that to yourself again?'

'Can't you keep your mouth shut just a little bit?'

'You think your sugar will be merciful for much longer?'

'You have no character. No will power! You're nothing!'

"I'm so good at that—a pro. I get mad at myself, promise myself this is the last time, and that tomorrow, I'm starting to really watch it."

I watched you, trying to feel, to understand.

I said; "I like your ability to differentiate between your types of eating. And, even more so, your ability to enjoy the good food to the fullest and find pleasure in it. I know, as you, yourself, realize, that this is not the eating that makes you so fat. Moreover, I think we would both sign off on 12 extra Kgs. of good and happy food as a perfect place for you.

"So, Tamar, let's talk to the sad food, the empty one, the one that comes in to substitute for something else. Something missing.

"Let's talk to it."

Tamar sometimes knows how to eat from a place of true pleasure. A place of no guilt. But a great deal of her eating is the kind accompanied by guilt and self-anger.

Most fat people don't allow themselves to enjoy eating even a bit. They are used to thinking that rich, tasty, pleasurable food is a "no-no," forbidden. In their experience, the list of forbidden foods is very long. It includes hamburgers, cakes, cereal, ice cream, steak, pasta with sauce, fine bread garnished with goat cheese and sun-dried tomato paste. They are used to so many prohibitions that if they only touch these foods, all hell breaks loose. And, honestly, how do you find balance in enjoying food, not feeling guilty, yet not experiencing uncontrollable eating binges?

It's not easy, I know.

I believe that if we eat tasty, gratifying food, dare to enjoy it—which most people find hard to do—perhaps then we can legitimize the pleasure. After all, if something is permissible, it doesn't arouse feelings of anger or worthlessness, hence, does not trigger binges.

Tamar, I see my role, not as someone who should tell you what to eat or not, but rather facilitate your ability to choose what to eat, when and how much. I will try to give you tools with which you can find out for yourself what you really want when you think you're hungry.

We won't create a guidebook for you to progress by. You will make up the guidebook based on the treatment you will undergo, your life situations, your feelings, and needs. That is, you will write your own book. Together we will try to find out what you feel while eating, what you truly need here and now, be it food or not. What is it that you truly need?

I once asked a patient to write her dream meal for me and describe in the most detailed fashion what her day would look like if she could eat all she wanted.

Francis wrote:

I would imagine this as the final meal before the Yom Kippur fast:[21] eat as much as possible in the shortest time possible. Stressful. I crave so many things, and I'm not sure I will have time to eat everything. If anything, I would like it to start in the morning and end late at night. But, to be efficient, let's start like this:

Coffee with milk in a large mug. Next to it, a crisp, fresh croissant full of butter, actually I feel like eating at least another four of those. Then a sweet yeast cake with raisins and crème pâtissière, yummy.

Then, actually before then, an omelet with thinly chopped toppings like bacon or ham with yellow cheese and sautéed onions. All fried in a pan with lots of butter for flavor. Next to the omelet, a vegetable salad, soft cream cheese, yellow cheese with toast and fresh bread (a fresh roll), then maybe another sunny-side-up with a fresh roll to "mop" up the yolk with. Then, or as I said before, the croissants.

About two hours later, I'll want a fresh baguette sandwich with butter and dry French Salami.

At lunchtime, which is actually right after the sandwich, I would eat a large portion of calamari with shrimp in garlic and wine sauce as well as another fried portion with a side sauce. A large dish of clams with a thin wine and cream sauce, escargot with bubbling butter, garlic, and parsley, and I would wipe off the sauce with a baguette. Yummy! Yummy!

I wouldn't mind a serving of spaghetti with seafood (the sauce with a little tomato and garlic), a serving of my lasagna recipe, sounds good to eat with the buried mushrooms, Béchamel sauce, cheese and turkey and the ground beef of course.

Out of this world!

---

[21]The final meal eaten before the Yom Kippur fast commences.

Moving on to a different "country." I'm dying to eat vegetable and shrimp tempura with like six Gyoza (That's it; I'm so hungry.).[22] For dessert, I want a tarte Tatin and another chocolate mousse cake with Brandy liquor and another slice of pecan pie and pear pie with fudge. A filo yeast cake with grated apples along with a chocolate cake, too.

I miss a French cake with tons of vanilla crème inside, filo dough from the outside, with the crème having some liqueur in it that adds a lot. The filo cake with almond crème filling would also be fun to eat. I miss that French cake.

Toward the evening, I want toast made from special bread (a large square slice with thin crust), spread with tons of butter, a little ketchup and a slice of turkey. For dessert, liquor candy in different flavors, sweet and sour, and those shaped like an alligator.

---

[22] A steamed meat dumpling with a heavenly dipping sauce.

November 1, 2000

Why do I put this guise over my body?

Where is that sensual woman hiding?

How I once used to enjoy looking in the mirror, examining my body, though not perfect, yet feminine, soft, smooth. I used to lounge on the beach, warming my body in the sun, as exposed as can be—enjoying it—entrusting it to others. It's so easy to find pleasure and be outward with the body. Why did I have to get so big? What am I running away from?

Why do I have to hide behind so much fat? What is it that I have to cover up, suppress so badly? It makes me so manly. The wide shoulders and the thick arms, the thick and short neck. A bull's nape. I look like a weightlifter. And this gigantic belly, hiding my entire self behind it. The entire woman that I am. You can always be patted on the back; no one's jealous; everyone loves you; you're not a threat; social, strong.

I'm fascinated by slender women, tall, light, how they bring forth their femininity and the surroundings immediately respond. Not everyone; true, femininity and sexiness is something you either have or you don't. It's not like you're necessarily attractive if you're thin. But if I were thin, I would be feminine, I would be attractive.

An entirely different life. Nothing is like the life of a fat body. Detached from itself, accumulating layers after layers, devising, deceitful, adulterous, bloated, heavy, numbed and defeated.

Humiliating, and everyone invades.

Being fat—a world unto itself.

It means always being apologetic. Everywhere you walk into, it's always your size first, no matter who you are. First, I apologize, then I make a joke about myself the first chance I get so that everyone is clear: I know, you know. Now that I've relieved you of your thoughts, speculations, whispers, you can relax. She talks about it, she laughs about it, it's not an issue anymore.

And when it's only men, I feel so worthless.

So valueless with male colleagues around.

Repulsive, disgusting, masculine, what do they think about me? "Why can't she do something about it?"

It's not intelligent to be fat.

It's gross, crude, common. All of our friends are preoccupied with their health, exercise, and take care, filled with self-discipline. And what about me?

I'm like a little girl that allows herself to let loose, without any ability to gather myself together and stick to a regime or a fitness lifestyle. One of health.

When I see a very fat man or child on the street, walking and stuffing some kind of junk food they bought into their mouth, I'm immediately overtaken by scorn and anger. How do they allow themselves?

How do I allow myself?

Whatever I put on myself, it's always gross.

No matter how much the clothes cost. It can't ever be elegant. I can't just throw something casual on.

Throwing something casual on is only for thin people.

When I go shopping at plus-size stores, I hate the fat customers who get excited about the colorful tents they're being offered. I also hate the saleswomen who flatter them.

"Oh, that looks amazing on you, it fits you so nicely." Everything is pathetic, so humiliating. I never want to be helped or consulted. I go in quickly, choose five to six items, try them on hastily, take a quick peek in the mirror closest to me. If there's a mirror in the dressing room, I don't even walk out.

I don't need anybody's advice, I don't want anyone to tell me how nice and elegant it is, because it's not. It's just a piece of fabric or huge sweater that covers up but can't hide anything.

Because nothing can be hidden.

It's just an illusion.

I pay quickly and rush out of the store.

That happens twice a year—winter and summer—I buy a few clothing items and buzz off.

If the next time I arrive at the store, the "oh so friendly" saleswomen remember me, ask for my name or what I do for a living, I never go back there.

I can't stand this familiarity. I don't want to feel at home. I don't want them to be nice to me. I don't want to be nice and polite.

I'm a sour-faced customer.

What are all those fat women smiling for?

What about?

Everyone always flatters me about my good taste. "I like your outfit."

What does it matter?

What does it matter if the nails are polished, or the face is all made up, when the foundation is so rotten, it's a waste of effort?

I live in shame and constant apology for my body.

My entire life is passing me through a screen.

I'm busy with my belly, being heavy, ashamed, different.

At the pool, I'm embarrassed to fit into a swimsuit, I don't want to be exposed, even though I love swimming so much.

In the water, you're light.

Swayed.

And in summer? Everything rubs against everything.

I hardly sweat, and I don't stink because I shower three times a day, scrubbing the fat from myself and always smelling good.

Always pulling my shirt over my belly when I sit down, thinking less will show. And if I walk places, I hope not to run into anybody.

At parties, when there's dancing, I'm never fully liberated because it looks so grotesque when someone so fat dances. It's like wanting to get a massage and being ashamed of your body. And trips? Forget about that, it's too hard.

It's taking up too much space between people, needing my own designated space, squeezing myself into seats at the movies, theater, dumping myself on Nadav because it would be embarrassing to do that to a stranger sitting on the other side, shrinking in embarrassment when people stare at me in disgust.

Forgive me for existing.
Why did I eat those soup croutons today?
Why did I mess up?

Ayelet, it's not another fluke, is it? It's already happening? Will it happen?
It's my time, right?
I would like to think it's not another bad attempt.
I would like to think, "This is the right time for me, that's why it's happening now." The beginning of my journey with you.
I would like to think that we have found each other, and perhaps something significant is going to happen to my eating. I have not accounted for my eating for such a long time, it's almost a new experience for me.
So many years.
It's new. To discuss, deal with what to eat—and what not.
Ayelet comments on important things, I know, and when she says them, they become real.
Like our eating habits at home. Why buy and cook fattening foods? I'm working on myself to prepare less and less fattening foods. To enjoy low-calorie things, eat only what gives me pleasure, not just gorge. It's so hard; I'm not skilled at it. I need Ayelet for coaching. I need to hear her repeat it over and over again.
She makes sure to say "we," "we ate," "we slipped," "we weighed." Joining me, how great.
Hand in hand. A true sense of togetherness.
She goes over my food lists with me, giving feedback to the point, what was good in each day and what was excessive; what

was a high-calorie day, what a harmless day is, and what a weight-loss day is.

Concrete, without blaming. Simple and to the point. Not reprimanding, non-judgmental. It mollifies the mythic notion that when you diet, you must give up everything, fast, suffer. Ayelet is accompanying me in my lifestyle, my eating habits, only suggesting how to introduce less food and more thought into my life.

So many of the other diets talk about pre-written food plans, meal times, set foods and your "optimal weight."

What Ayelet offers makes it livable.

It's not all or nothing; you can eat and enjoy yourself and still lose weight. You can negotiate with the food. Try to cut your losses. Losses of weight. Lose the food but win.

I think Ayelet is mainly teaching me that I can introduce control and order into this eating chaos. Eating doesn't have to be chaotic, as she calls it. Keeping track like this forces me to start managing my life with regard to food.

With Ayelet, the weight is not the issue.

Sometimes, you don't get weighed, if I don't want to or if Ayelet thinks it's not right for me.

Sometimes, she offers not to weigh me even if she thinks I lost weight. Because according to my eating journal, I don't deserve to lose weight, and it doesn't even matter what the scale says.

What's important for Ayelet is mainly that I was in touch with myself during the week, aware, able to give up, or better yet, able to choose what to give up.

Whether I'm able to get out of the compulsive patterns of seeing food and instantly consuming it or thinking about food and immediately finding it.

The important thing is facilitating awareness as with many other things.

Not just the food.

To be in touch with myself and eat less.

Ayelet wants it all and fast, while I want it all and slow. But she's with me. She's definitely with me. She's completely there for me as a therapist, able to contain me and mainly unafraid of me, which is something very new for me.

I'm preoccupied with my relationship with her, but I'm also willing to follow her even though I don't know what it means for me. I haven't done anything real for thirteen years, ever since Mai was born. Be patient with me, Ayelet, I know nothing about myself, and I'm forty-one today.

The meta-cognition of my eating is only on a theoretical level, not on the practical level, in true coping. When you asked what I could really give up, I gave up on more eating tonight. I let a thought into my head that said, "You've eaten enough today. You're not really hungry. At least not for food." A new experience for me.

This morning, at work, I succeeded. And in the evening, around the table, I ate chaotically. Where am I?

At the very beginning. But, Tamar, you've never experienced such a therapeutic approach to your eating problem—never. It's like nothing you've ever done.

You're in a different place today. And part of your depression is engraved in the fat that you're drowning in. And, for the first time in years, with all this sabotage and self-talk of yours, you might just want to live another life that exists in you, a life of lightness, health, precision.

Sometimes you're old, letting everything slide underneath you for the sake of slumber, dipping under the diffusion of oblivion.

Being fat is like being handicapped.

It screams, it accosts my consciousness, it's with me every single moment. It's thinking how everyone is looking at me in a crowded elevator, afraid that it may not carry the weight and get stuck.

You hardly carry yourself, developing old people's illnesses: cancer, diabetes, high blood pressure, knee pain. You're only forty. You could have been light, healthy, beautiful and strong, instead of a tired, wilted sack.

I'm telling you, again and again, asking, begging, "Don't do it 'semi.' Don't do it partially, or almost." Damn it, go for it, go with yourself—go!

The same was with Yael.

All fire. Gushing, cascading golden curls.

At times it seemed like everything was spilling over, about to burst in intensities of benevolence, love, and passion.

I met her years ago; another diet, another weight loss process.

She lost weight, left, came back, gained weight and then lost some, and for a moment there, it seemed like we broke the code, found the key. But the cards got shuffled frequently. Every emotional uproar, every man that entered her life or even touched it, made her disoriented. Her entire power would be devoured into a world where sex, partnership, and femininity played a key role.

Yael.

A successful career woman in her mid-thirties, surrounded by family and wonderful girlfriends.

A life full of action, interest and progress.

A knowing, demanding, decisive woman, yet:

Searching.

Maddened.

Getting lost.

The golden curls cascading, misleading, deceiving;

Her?

For years, she didn't know emotional tenderness or experience a real, fulfilling and reciprocating relationship;

she was always in a state of missing, of failing to discover. A worldly woman, so alive and yet so alone in it.

Sometimes we attributed the eating to the unfulfilled powers in her. Her fat encompasses her sexuality, her desires. And the eating, what does it involve?

Lust, pleasure. She has all these, big time, just like everything else about her is big. That's how it is. She eats, gives, touches, loves in abundance that only she knows.

And eventually, he arrived, albeit late, and somewhat surprisingly, he did.

And she was riled, as I have never seen her before, swept into this tempting, consuming relationship.

Tasting, chewing, taking pleasure. Flavors her palate had not known before; had not felt or touched.

And was succulent, luring, like quicksand.

And she, deeply immersed in the couple, only seldom in solitude, after waiting for this union for so long. Waiting so long until it morphed into this new thing, into the other.

She smiled and gained weight.

Absorbed and bloated.

Felt the union and grew to a size I had never seen her in before.

The fat spoke out what she did not know to begin with. And the fat said all that she felt but didn't want to see. She ate, took pleasure, and paid the price.

She ate, until satiation, and wanted more.

The relationship watered and fertilized, but also unraveled and unstitched.

And she got lost in it. For herself?

And the kilograms piled. Layer upon layer, weighted and burdening, as was the relationship and the union. Something there needed the sheltering of fat. Something in her needed the food.

Was it defiance?

Protecting her boundaries?

It's hard for me to say, but I was no doubt surprised.

I was hoping it would be different; that she would be filled by the union and not the food; that she wouldn't need to put such clear boundaries; that she wouldn't need the eating and that sex would fill what was missing. I was hoping that the void would be filled with feeling, lust and desires of the kind she had not known.

That it would be different.

But it transpired otherwise.

There were moments when it seemed she would do anything to survive in this relationship.

But the union demanded huge concessions from her. She was consumed by it, and perhaps she needed to expand so much in order to stay in it. And perhaps, those concessions required the banal compensation of food.

Because that union led her to entirely different places than those she wanted.

She was forced to leave her new, comfortable home and move to a small, old and somewhat dilapidated house, very different from the luxurious neighborhood she was living in. And she didn't have an intimate corner for herself in that house. She didn't feel like she belonged, but she tried, she made an effort.

Every night, she stood in the kitchen, cooking dinner. She put a lot of thought into the ingredients, the flavors, the quality. This in itself was foreign to her, but she was so keen, and she saw how happy and cheerful her partner was, so she gave more. She was so eager to pamper, to shower with affection. With a flower, a small gift, love. And he enjoyed it and took it, and wanted more all the time.

The gaps between them began to show as she found it hard to accept his unwillingness to make an effort on a professional level. There were times when she felt "better," more accomplished, more successful. And, in order to conceal the differences in quality and success, he would downgrade and humiliate her.

Yael was an executive in a successful company, with top professional achievements and highly regarded in her areas of expertise. And he found it hard to match that and prove himself. From his weak standpoint, he hurt her where she cared the most——in the bedroom, with her sexuality. He would bluntly question her ability to satisfy him. He would devalue her for not being attractive enough, for not having a "perfect figure."

And she gained weight.

There was a tone of defiance in her obesity. Like a defense wall. "You won't decide on or manage my body. I won't change for you. I'm only yours up to here, and from here on, I'm mine. And you can't go beyond this point."

Perhaps the eating involved sadness for the fact that this union wasn't reaching the level she hoped to meet and feel? Or perhaps, there was anger in it toward him, who was trying to doubt her sexuality, who tried to touch those places that were taboo.

And then, she covered up her femininity in another layer of fat, as if giving him a justifiable reason. He messed up many of her ways, shuffled many of her cards, and she became consumed as well as consuming herself. He triggered in her an uncertainty and insecurity about her femininity. He made her feel worthless.

So much so that she became tired, defeated, and sought out to defend herself, her life, her desires and her genuine needs.

That was painful.

That was hard.

But putting on 10 Kgs. in such a short time indicated to her that something in that relationship wasn't good for her or truly nurturing and loving. That she was not receiving the real affection she was looking for and that she was using the food to make up for what was missing. And that surely couldn't be the way.

And then, she broke up with him; and the solitude was scary, cold and desolate. It brought her back to her beautiful, elegant home, to her girlfriends who were angry about the "oppressive boyfriend," who, though hurtful, at least kept her warm and embraced.

And I watch from the sidelines, sometimes feeling, sometimes knowing, a little sad, and perhaps sorry, but knowing that for now, she had chosen what is good for her.

Two years later, she has dropped 14 Kgs. She sticks to her physical exercise, which has performed miracles in her body. But above all, she simply looks and feels wonderful.

She is at the beginning of a new relationship, which fills her heart with love, and continues to take a great interest in her work and in the world around her.

But I believe she is mostly happy with being herself.

November 7, 2000

Ayelet. I manage to breathe next to her, remain open, for the most part, in this constricted place. I arrive constricted but manage to stay and to open up.

Is she connected?

Are her body and spirit connected?

Is she connected to creation?

Everything is easier when you're connected to creation.

Nothing happens without reason, and everything happens only when we allow it, and when it's time to choose.

Just like today, when I managed to find my center, and feel at home, softly, excitedly. My center, which is as wide as my lips, moving from my lips along my entire body, dividing and connecting it. That is where my spark is. That is where light is created and absorbed.

When I'm able to connect to my center, I feel at home, I'm present. Not numbed, not vacant. I breathe in deeply, feeling the knots in me come undone and that there is room for my spark to ascend and descend with no interruptions. Then I can connect to what I truly need.

Not running away. Not being different. Not being almost.

Being present.
Me.

Just as more and more layers were revealed to me today, and creation peeked.

I breathe the light into me and am open today as I have not been in a long time. And I can touch love. And I'm home, in my center. A new essence, kind and benevolent.
That is how I can start to really touch my fat self.
I don't struggle, I don't fight, I begin to allow thought and awareness to enter my eating. I see what I eat, not like a blind person, not feeling my way in the dark, with the debate going on in my head, "Yes or no, maybe later?" there is thought. Sometimes, even a plan. Sometimes.
I am on the verge of beginning, but perhaps for the first time, I'm not afraid to lose. Not afraid to lose the diet, because I'm not dieting.
I have less compulsive thoughts. Sometimes, I'm able to feel less compelled to eat.
Many times, I get a thought stuck in my head about a certain kind of food. I can be in the middle of reading a book, doing house chores, with my kids, with Nadav, in some home situation. And the thought gets stuck and doesn't leave. And it paralyzes me. And then, like a robot, I walk to the kitchen, preparing what it was that stuck in my head, and instead of stuffing that thought, I now have food stuffed in me. And then, when the thought lets go, I have a momentary break, immediately followed by a guilty conscience.

And in this entire vicious cycle of compulsive thinking, there is no room to break in and let a little light, a little air, a little life in.

It's a dead, lifeless process.

A stifling, exhausting process.

I'm a little girl; I constantly need coaching. It seems to be the only way it works. I now realize that for the last two years, I've been searching for someone to coach me, practically and emotionally.

How everything happens in its due course.

It couldn't have happened earlier.

The place of eating comes from the id, the passion, the animal in me, the deepest, most primal places before I ever became a person. I feel, I let myself go wild with my desire, only with food, because here it's least dangerous. Any other desire is dangerous. So, the fat protects, shields.

Like I told Ayelet, when I lose control and can't get a thought in, it's like a screen goes up, impenetrable, and my head empties, there is only body and need, body and need and no intervention.

Ayelet has good, productive ideas.

As soon as you come home, something hot, or precut vegetables are fun, cherry tomatoes, pickles. An intervention using a toothbrush at night is nice.

Because after I brush my teeth at night, the kitchen is closed, and there is no legitimacy to eat.

Today, I finished a huge meal, and I still ate chocolate and a granola bar. How unnecessary. And the whole idea of brushing my teeth was in my head, but I didn't succeed in doing it. I must have a little sabotage; it's a habit of mine. But I will give it up, without fighting, when I allow it.

The fear of losing weight is the fear of disappearing. That's what Meir says. What will happen if I'm no longer fat? What would it be like to live an easier life?

The truth is I don't know what it means to be a thinner forty-one-year-old woman. It's not who I was when I was twenty.

But that's the only thing I can think about. That single picture, that single image. Me at about twenty-five years. It was the last year I looked good and felt good with my body. And, back then, it was dangerous for me. That body mainly got me into trouble.

If I could invite a new thought, "Forty-one-year-old," maybe then I would be able to imagine myself a light forty-one-year-old, not fat; maybe then I would stop being afraid.

Because maybe it's no longer dangerous at the age of forty-one. And if I lose weight significantly, wrinkles will appear just as they do on my girlfriends' faces. And at forty-one, looking good is surely less dangerous than at twenty-five.

I know for certain that my sense of reality will be stronger, and I will be less isolated from the world.

It's actually an invigorating thought.

But what if my intensities are less confined?

Maybe they will subside, fade, calm down, find peace?

Or maybe this is all just a fantasy.

Maybe, like all fat people, I'm also blaming my fat for all the suffering, and when the fat dissolves, I'll be left with the suffering?

What will the excuse be then?

I'm really not feeling good about Ayelet's trip, mainly because of the writing.

I guess it will be hard to keep up the writing if we don't follow up on it for so many days.

But there is a lesson here. I think the lesson is me— tackling those pages on my own, the ability to give myself some feedback, not too judgmental.

One of the things that is happening to me now is that I'm able to be less judgmental of myself on the subject that I so disparage—my obesity.

In general, I look back at how judgmental and cynical I have been toward myself, and now most of that cynicism is left in my poetry, and I hurt myself less.

The journaling is becoming something more than just about obesity.

What I give is what I'll get; I know that very well, and I'm the creator.

I feel like air is coming in, rays of light, of creation, are starting to seep in between me and my fat.

Maybe I'm starting to separate, to stay home, in my own center, separating myself from the heaviness. Maybe I'll allow myself to be light.

Maybe this is the transference with which I can soar high and be an elevated soul.

Connect to the spirit inside me— the divine spark. Maybe I'll find the spark within me and learn to take my consciousness on a journey where I can find the light, not just the chaos. The simple, clear light—the divine—in all that is inside me.

Maybe I'll find simplicity. And then, I'll stop searching.

I could be more spirit and less body.

Ayelet, how will I read you everything that I've been studying for three years in workshops and sessions with Meir? How will I explain? But I won't explain, and whatever you can take, you'll take.

It's important that I check with myself how I feel when I'm eating compulsively, and that I can only do with Ayelet.

This week with Ayelet was good.

November 14, 2000

Tamar, what is it about you that entices me, challenges me, makes me want to succeed?

I ask myself, is this how I feel toward all of my patients, or is it something special about you?

And I know this is something that characterizes my entire work approach. I often have the tendency to want to please the patient. I see his suffering, his hardship, and I believe with all my heart that he could feel differently if he only dropped some of his weight, so then I am dominated by my strong desire for him to reach that particular place where he will feel better.

I am aware that these needs are my own and that I project them onto my patients as if I can want something on their behalf. Besides, why am I so certain I know what they want? This notion that I must help the person help himself hangs very heavy on me and maybe even on my patients, who may be attempting to please me.

The same goes for you, Tamar, I want on your behalf, I make an effort on your behalf.

And what is this success I keep mentioning? Is it the success of losing weight, or feeling good about yourself, with your body? Or perhaps learning to talk to your inner hunger that controls you and drowns you in a sea of endless eating?

Is success the journey itself or its outcome?

I think for me, success would be your success, Tamar, reaching a place where you feel good with who you are, with your body and your eating habits. This is an internal place that is solely yours. Only you can feel it. It's not a number, not a weight.

This good place is a physical and emotional sensation you can feel and internalize. You will know it when you reach it. It's a place you can maintain without abstinence or starvation, but with mindful, thoughtful eating. Therefore, this place cannot be measured by absolute values; it is a relative figure that is individually suited for you, your personality, your weight history and the current period in your life.

This success also depends on other factors: On the ability to persist in a framework, regardless of the week's events; to continue journaling even on lopsided, chaotic days; to feel the hunger and try to determine where it stems from, whether it is truly physical hunger or maybe emotional hunger. And, if it is emotional, to stay with it without numbing it, eat from a mindful, thoughtful place instead of an automatic, overpowering one.

And mostly, the ability to be. With yourself. Not with the substitutes.

You can compare this treatment to a building under construction.

137

Day after day, for many months, as you walk past that building, it seems like nothing is happening, layer after layer, and it's as if nothing is being erected. No progress made. Until one day, as you walk past that same construction site, all of a sudden, the building is there. Impressively standing. So is the therapeutic process. It is slow, drawn out, sometimes seeming like it's going nowhere. The changes are almost indiscernible, and the patient may think that nothing is happening. But, in reality, processes are taking place all the time. Some are invisible, unconscious, until the patient experiences, digests, internalizes and discovers these abilities inside him. The ability to accept change, to feel it and enjoy it. And then, all of a sudden, as if by surprise, he is in a new, different place.

And where am I?

Sometimes, while busy trying to understand your eating, I observe my own, trying to understand the difference, characteristics, and my needs.

And I am not devoid of passions and desires for food. For instance, I know I'm crazy about good bread and yellow cheese, or shrimp in tomato and mint sauce. Both simple and refined food; I find it hard to resist chocolate yeast cakes, but a plate of vegetables can be just as inviting. So, it's hard to say that I don't gain weight because I don't have incurable needs and desires. But I think that over the years, despite or perhaps due to the genetics of obesity in my family over the generations, I have developed self-control techniques that enable me to have a real dialogue with my eating. Thus, even my eating binges are conscious and chosen. My need to feel good with my body is strong in a way that has enabled me to develop an empathetic dialogue with my food.

And it's not that easy. But the physical weightiness is even harder for me to bear.

About twenty-two years ago, during a long backpacking trip, we took a break in Australia, a place that was a huge discovery for me as an Israeli back then. An abundance of temptations. We were sprawled by the poolside. I distinctly remember the mango and the Kit-Kat bars I gorged on pleasurably, out of sheer addiction to the taste, and a desire that knew no satisfaction.

The outcome was 8 extra kilograms, changing to a bigger pants size and a lot of heaviness.

And it's not that I didn't like the intoxicating, overpowering addiction. But more than I liked it, I hated the sense of estrangement from myself and my body. And I guess for me that was stronger and helped me manage my inner dialogue.

Two months later, after a trip to Papua New Guinea and the Philippines, it seemed like I had dropped all of it.

But that is my story.

We are different from each other, and we don't necessarily have to, or can be, shaped into identical molds.

Part of understanding the world of obesity is perhaps accepting the difference and seeing the beauty in it.

This should not be interpreted as if I believe obesity is something that should be outright legitimized. But I definitely believe and know that utopic thinness cannot control us. The only goal should be to achieve one's private place of well-being. And this place is different from person to person. Tamar, I would like to suggest that you try to reach your own place, one that will accept you and one you can accept.

December 3, 2000

It's exactly a month since I opened this journal.

Whenever I open it, I immediately open a window to the sorrow that fills me and my throat tightens. This is the first time I've admitted it to myself. Yes, it's so painful.

I didn't know that being fat hurts me so much. That's always been the problem, it's always been with me; I carry this awareness in every moment of my life, but I've never touched the pain like I'm doing now.

It's a discovery for me. I didn't know how much it hurt me.

It hurts on a physical level. I open the journal, and it hurts in my throat, in my lungs, in my spine, the pain just pours, and I don't know what to do with it except cover it up with more and more flab.

Maybe some of the scars in my hyper-sensitive, unnerving life are covered in a veil of numbing flab, and then it hurts less, leaving just the sensation, just the habit.

When I imagine myself looking good, it's always in a sensual or sexual connotation. It's like I can't just go to work looking good or enjoy dressing up. It's as if looking good and feeling good, healthy and attractive with my body can only be sexual or sensual.

How scary.

Ayelet left after we read what we wrote to each other.

Excitement and pain, lots of intimacy and forgiveness, how scary.

It's the first time I read what I wrote, and just like that, I give in. At once, everything comes out, opens, exposed before Ayelet. I give in to her so easily.

She untangles my insides and stretches it out. It was all there, it just needed to be read.

I'm surprised at how much my intimate life was revealed to her.

I actually never exposed myself to anyone in this way. No one knows my inner world fat world. This whole game of openness, sincerity, is in the parts I choose, not the dark parts.

But opening all that up to Ayelet was scary.

And she, with a lot of courage, honesty, unafraid, bringing herself into some parts of the therapy. It's powerful for me, and interesting, and I wasn't alarmed by Ayelet's part.

I wanted to touch her, but you can't touch. You can't touch Ayelet.

There is a transparent, invisible curtain she hides herself behind as a therapist and as a person. I never hugged or touched her, which is something I usually do so easily.

A curtain made of clear crystal fibers blocks the way. And what happens if you put your hand through the curtain? Will it melt? Will it vanish?

If I touch her cold, skinny, pale hand with my warm, soft hand, will she burst? Retract? Dodge it?

Maybe Ayelet can't take that?

And the tables turn, because, in this complex relationship, she gives of herself in a measured, calculated way. And I'm used to the total opposite relationships in which the other gives in, opens up, needs, attaches and I tak it slowly. It takes me years, if at all, and even then, it's at my pace, and only partially.

All this has made me panic, so I didn't write, and so when Ayelet left, I didn't stop eating. I feel that the pace in which I keep in my eating, in my body, in daily life, is my true pace. This is on top of my tremendous difficulty in truly being able to bring some thought into my eating.

I write, but the instinctive response, for the most part, wins. And suddenly, I notice that I already ate five olives from the jar; shaved off here and there a few slices of bread from the freezer popped in the microwave, and they're already covered with butter and avocado, a few small spoons of green tahini sauce, and finally a few small spoons of jelly. By the time I stop, 400–500 calories have been consumed by the giant body without me even feeling I had eaten anything.

I deal with it; I don't give up; I hardly go wild for full days at a time.

I'm not really succeeding, but at least I know what I'm eating. Sometimes, I'm able to plan, cook with less oil for the guests, and when I come home from work, I eat something warm and filling without a lot of calories.

Ayelet Kalter

I don't even have eating habits; nothing is planned. Just like many other aspects of my life, they simply happen, one thing leads to another.

So, say I start doing some chore at home, like cooking, and I go upstairs to get something, I'll have to clean the room I walked into, and usually on the way down, I run into some dirty laundry, so I take it downstairs, totally forgetting I started to cook.

At work, I manage a lot, but I'm not organized or planned enough. There too, one thing leads to another, and I could really be more efficient.

When I'm on my own, time flies by without much accomplished. Or if I run errands, I plan where I start, but then find myself in places and stores I never even intended to visit.

It's like I whiz by things and then stop, only to whiz by again.

I need to start from the top. But not talk about it, like, "Oh, how great I am" at something. Now it's important for me to listen to Ayelet's advice. Say it to myself but really loud and then try to do it, internalize and act.

I need these crutches from Ayelet right at the start, all the time. But when I finally stand in front of hot pastry, sometimes I can tell myself, even aloud, that it's bad, it's fattening, it's bad for the sugar, it's calorically "expensive" like Ayelet says.

It's humiliating how weak I am in this area. With knowing more or less how many calories are in everything.

And I also need a lot of food to fill me up.

And I eat fast, too. How?! How am I going to make it?! It brings me back to the pain.

I used to enjoy hanging out only with boys—men.

This is where I felt most comfortable, most direct, most exciting, the least betraying.

I mainly had friends and acquaintances, boys, men.

Today, I find myself embarrassed when I'm in the company of men only, even the closest, most intimate friends. I find it uncomfortable, and my awkwardness stems from my size and discomfort with my body, which is all of a sudden so amplified when I'm only with men.

I immediately feel threatened, can't have anybody touch me or come close to me.

If the situation calls for couples—at a social gathering with friend couples—then I touch, come close, hug, feel. I can hug her and him only when they're in a couple. I can't even handle something that resembles tension between the sexes.

I can't handle it.

In the cold December, we descended into this darkness.
There were rows of graves that collapsed
Like dominos tumbling on each other.
And hairy muddy holes gaped, and from all of them
Peeked effervescent gray potbellies of live dough
And worms had already infested the potbellies
And it closed again, and opened again
An oil stain. So when they flatten me with a press,
This is all that will be left.

December 10, 2000

Tamar,

I embarked on this journey with mixed feelings of curiosity, dread, challenge and fear of failure.

And indeed, we arrived at the first pothole in the road, which was perhaps expected, but like any obstacle, raised questions, a little confusing and mainly intimidating.

You and I were thrown into a fairly long time-out since I was away on work for two weeks.

I traveled to a conference in Philadelphia. A fascinating conference about feministic approaches to treating eating disorders and trauma. I traveled both for sightseeing and professional enrichment, but whatever the reason may be, any hiatus or time-out in the therapeutic continuum may be a cause for trouble. Especially for those people who are in the midst of undergoing treatment. They are sometimes shaken, wandering lost, as if their crutches were taken away from them.

And so, it happened to you.

You walked in, big, huge and present — but tired and slightly defeated.

There was a thick veil of disappointment in your expression.

"I waited for you, I missed you," you said.

I left.

And the boundaries melted.

You didn't manage to internalize them. They were outside of you. Not yours.

And everything became liquid-like, diffused.

And you drowned, Tamar.

Simple as that.

You got carried away and consumed by the stormy sea of tempting foods.

And food went back to ruling your life belligerently. And it's not like this outbreak had pleasure, satisfaction, and excitement.

It filled you, but it was guzzling to the point of disgust, oblivion and numbness of passion and feeling. This eating had an exhausting, paralyzing heaviness. Like a signal, "Look, I'm drowning." You disappeared, disappeared from yourself. You stopped writing in your eating journals, you stopped asking questions.

You simply ate.

And it hurt you, it singed you, but it was stronger than you. You felt, knew, but couldn't stop.

And I, who left, was afraid of that place.

Because we are only at the start of the journey. I gave you my hand, and you agreed to take it. We began to build the trust between us. You said you gave into it to a certain degree. I offered you paths to walk on. I was there for you every week.

And I left. When for you, everything was only starting.

Three months, a delicate time frame.

Time off hinders a process, especially when it's in the inception stages. I try to choose my absences very carefully, out of an honest attempt to consider my patients' needs. But, despite it all, many times these breaks pose a real problem.

I felt your distress to the fullest, Tamar. This is where I, too, feel the intensity of the task I have taken on myself. I have a tendency to extend my hand, caress, embrace, be nurturing and identify. But I must be wary.

Not to identify, I tell myself; identification will be a hindrance, it can delay, affix, intensify the fall. I must gather myself and remain at arm's reach. A therapeutic distance from which I can lead you to better places for yourself. I want the hand I offer you to be brave, one that can be leaned against a little, but not hang on it. A hand that will mostly give strength and power and will restore your faith in yourself and your abilities.

You were already there, Tamar, there is no reason you cannot succeed again.

Just carry on.

And that is what I tried to do.

It hurt me, I felt heavy and sad. I understood the suffering you experienced. I felt the strain of falling into the menacing abyss again. But, despite the empathy I felt, and despite my strong desire to shield and contain, I tried to challenge you anew, to elevate and mainly to bring you to regain your motivation and commitment to yourself and to your body.

As an additional exercise to the usual journaling, I asked you to start to converse with the inner hunger controlling you. To try to think for a moment before you fall into your automatic eating behavior, and ask yourself what is this behavior supposed to address at that moment. What is in it for you? Real hunger? Boredom? Emptiness? Compensation? I know it's a hard and intimidating task since it involves deep and probing self-talk.

And indeed, by keeping an eating journal and identifying the stimuli that trigger your binges, you have begun to develop awareness to your tempestuous eating world. You observed thoughts, feelings, and hunger.

I posed questions that I wanted you to ask yourself:

"How hungry are you really during and around a binge?"

"Do you abstain from food in the hours or days before a binge?"

"Can you identify in yourself a state of increased eating followed by the start of a controlled diet?"

I asked that you try to write your feelings around hunger and its role controlling your binges. "Try to examine and discover the positive and negative feelings that affect your eating."

"What did you feel before, during and after the binge?"

"Do your binges arouse feelings of pleasure and entertainment in you?"

"Does the notion that you feel bad after a binge perhaps create feelings of self-punishment?"

You should also examine your thoughts.

"What thoughts affect your eating?"

"What do you think before, during and after the binge?"

"Do you binge in order to divert the focus from negative thoughts to thoughts about food?"[23]

After you examined yourself using these questions, you were rather terrified, at least that is what I felt. You truly realized that a great deal of your life, thoughts, and feelings is motivated by food, feels and is satisfied through it.

"Ayelet, I feel like there isn't a point on this list of questions I can't relate to.

"I have to admit, I don't really think before my binges. What for? I won't be able to prevent them. They show up in almost every emotional state. When I'm happy and sad, angry or anxious. Only seldom do I find myself in an emotional state that will prevent me from eating. Especially if the food is available and tempting. And you know what? Even if it's not available, I'll find my way to it.

"I notice that I remember trips according to the restaurants we ate in and the types of dishes, their taste, and specialty. I longingly recall amazing eating places that combined delicacies with ambiance.

"Besides, Ayelet, you're really not with it, and you don't get it. There is nothing that can stop me from craving food. Any instance like that would require restraint and some sort of giving up.

---

[23] Agras, Stewart W. & Robin F. Apple. *Overcoming Eating Disorders. A Cognitive-Behavioral Treatment for Bulimia Nervosa and Binge Eating Disorders.* Graywind Publication Incorporated, 1997. Therapist Guide Client Workbook.

"You talk about thoughts. Of course, I hate my body, my fat, my huge belly and my double chin. But when the food stands before me, who remembers, who knows? Everything gets garbled up inside me and summons me to go for it.

"And when I go for it, I got lost very quickly. I lead my feelings and thoughts astray in a sea of food and pleasures. So, what if these are short-term pleasures; they have so much sensuality and enjoyment. And you want me to give those up?

"And then, who remembers the ailment, the pain, and the heaviness. Instant gratification is the only thing I see before me. And I can't think of anything that would prevent me from having that eating binge because there are no thoughts at that moment. They only come up after the binge or toward the end of it. And then, of course, all hell breaks loose. Because I'm really good at beating myself up. And I'm an expert on promising this will be the last time.

"That is why I'm usually around 110 Kgs."

And I? I listen, know and find it hard to help.

And Hila writes in her journal:

Today I ate more than 3,000 calories.
I'm so tired.
I ate myself sick. I saw one of my dieticians on TV and I started crying.
I'm just crying.
I had a very humiliating conversation with Rony.
Don't you have any limits?

I mustn't call him at all tomorrow or the next day.
Am I crazy?
What does it mean to be crazy?
I just humiliated myself.
And he doesn't respond.
God
Good night
I'm so tired.

Tamar, beyond the difficult dialogue you had with yourself, I wanted to try to give you a few tools to cope with the thoughts that control your eating.

Step 1: Try to identify the specific problem that can trigger you to go into uncontrollable eating (For example, "I don't have any plans for tonight, I'm in a horrible mood, and I feel bad about myself, and the only way out for me is to shove a bar of chocolate.")

Step 2: Try to raise all the possibilities of handling the problem without evaluating or judging. And using that to try to choose the best way for you without self-criticism (examples, guzzle chocolate in order to cope with the real feelings, allow myself to eat chocolate without losing control, leave the current situation, go for a walk, call a friend, clean the house, answer letters or take care of piling paperwork).

Step 3: Evaluate the efficiency and practicality of all the possibilities raised.

Step 4: Choose one option that seems most proper.

Step 5: Try to follow the effect of the option chosen on the binge.

Step 6: Try to draw conclusions from the process so that you can use it in other situations.[24]

You said, "Wow...what an overload...you really think I can do something with all the information you dropped on me? It seems so contrived, unrealistic, unauthentic. You really think I can think before each bite I put in my mouth? You really think that there are steps to my inner dialogue with food? I see and eat. I feel and eat. Who is even free to ask, examine, choose? What are you talking about?

"What control? What inner dialogue?

"Ayelet, wake up. Look at me. Do I look to you like someone in control?

"Do I look to you like someone who can restrain herself?"

I responded with, "Wow...

"How intense...

"Tamar, Tamar, don't be alarmed. I'm not trying to shape you into some behavioral molds or rules. I'm just trying to make you aware of their existence.

"I want to bring you closer to yourself a little. That's all.

"You decide what to do and how. I'm by your side, but you choose what to do with it. I'm not trying to "drop" any plan or assignments on you. I just felt the need to lay down another perspective before you."

---

[24]Agras, *Overcoming Eating Disorders.*

Another stage.

You debated, hesitated, but I think you dared take this complex mission having a discussion with your inner hunger.

And you walked out big, huge. Unique as always.
And you walked out with your head held high!

December 13, 2000

Inner hunger.

What is inner hunger?

Ayelet gave me a mission to have a discussion with my inner hunger. A didactic mission. Having a discussion reminds me of school. Of my parents being summoned to discuss how unruly I was. I remember my poor mother walking up the road that led to my high school to discuss how I didn't fulfill my potential, how I didn't study, that I was disruptive and rude. A bad girl.

Hunger is not something you can discuss anything with; unger doesn't understand words.

Hunger is a hole—a cunning hole of solitude.

Hunger is a cave or better yet a tunnel that is constantly inside, on the left side of the body or the soul. And this tunnel is moist, dark, moldy and always inviting to crawl into, lie on your back, curled up in humidity that slowly becomes warmer and steamy.

There, you slowly detach from the outside world, as its noises gradually fade.

And you remain there, sucked into yourself, into that big hole in yourself, where you come face to face with the shiniest, gleaming solitude.

I don't know how to exit this tunnel by myself. What pulls me out of there is the life taking place outside. My family, my work, my friends.

The outside reality that summons me to be that jostles me out of the tunnel until the next time.

This is what you want me to talk to?

Who can handle that?

It's not like you know how to talk to your hunger, Ayelet.

Maybe you try to satisfy it with other things.

You cheat your hunger. You try to pacify it by being constantly busy and by incessantly consuming culture.

Whenever I arrive at your clinic, there's always a new book or CD.

You're an obsessive consumer of culture.

Your hunger just doesn't show on your body.

You know what? My hunger is more honest than yours.

At least mine tries honestly to fill itself with food.

Talk to your hunger, Ayelet.

I don't want to talk at all.

I have no wheeling and dealing with it.

It's just there.

All the time.

Waiting.

December 19, 2000

You didn't exactly address the tasks. You weren't able to invest real attention in them that would lead to action on your part, or to the discovery of a genuine insight on your own eating. I asked myself why? Perhaps it's the overload of questions that threatened you? Or perhaps my requests came too early in the treatment?

I sensed your ambivalence in every step of the way. Your difficulty in letting go of every gram.

You cooperate, but you don't.

You do a little and then stop for a little.

The process is excruciatingly slow. After all, with an overweight such as yours, the kilograms should be pouring off of you, so to speak.

But here, everything is drawn out and encumbered. And it's not the physical difficulty in losing weight. It's the difficulty in giving up these protective walls, and this passionate, wild eating style. The oddity of thinking of yourself as not huge.

I feel you taking cautious steps, testing.

On previous diets, you would lose weight in a storm. Whereas here, everything is more hesitant, questioning.

Without realizing, small, yet significant changes are being made. There are no more binges, hardly any mindless eating, a lot more planning and awareness and especially, surrender.

The changes are hidden at times. And the weight loss also is slow. It mostly involves loss of bloating. Your general feeling is better. And, interestingly, the environment, as always, responds. And it helps you, you say; it rewards you.

A few positive feedbacks. People say you look better. No one says you lost weight so far, but everyone notices that something has softened in you.

"And that's nice," you say, smiling shyly.

I feel the inner conflict taking place inside you very well. I have no doubt you want to succeed, and I have no doubt it's hard for you. Not only is it hard to give up the large quantities of food or the type of food you choose to eat. Losing weight is something deeper. In your experience, in the personal journey you are undergoing, you talk about self-sabotage, destruction. About forces stronger than yourself that control you, as it were.

In reality, Tamar, I feel that you are stronger. Your main hurdle is your struggle with yourself, your commitment to an inner dialogue. You can't do it without an inner dialogue. I believe it can prevent you from unconscious eating.

Perhaps what is so hard for you, Tamar, as it would be for any person, is to begin to interact with those genuine places.

It is an inner dialogue that takes on a different form and version with each person. But its very existence sheds light from a different angle on food and its role in our life.

The following lines, taken from Gili's journal, will illustrate my point:

December 10, 2000

I think I can describe exactly what you look like.

Mainly because you're asleep now. Small, huddled, black, but still there.

Like a germ that can spread at any moment, if it only spends enough time alone with me.

Tiny-ish, but alive and breathing, your own entity. I'm supposed to decide when you show up or not.

You're asleep now. You've slept the whole day. Your color has turned grayish somewhat faded. When I was at the clothing store with Michal, looking at myself in the mirror, I saw you jumping on the opportunity and taking control of me all at once.

Luckily, I wasn't alone.

Good thing I stayed with Michal.

It depressed you, I know.

Just then you got that gray of yours, and I didn't want to be alone with you because then you grow so strong. You intensify. I feel like you'll always be with me. I want to get rid of you for good. I don't know if it's possible.

December 11, 2000

Today you lead.

You've taken on a new form.

Today you're a space inside me. Not just my stomach. My entire body.

To the tips of my fingers.

I think you know I'm seriously considering getting rid of you soon, and that makes you panic. You grow stronger. I may not get rid of you so fast, but I can make you shrink, I can make you pretty faded, you know.

I can fight and eat like a normal person for a whole week and surround myself with people I love, and you weaken, but you're still there.

Small, but there.

Always waiting for an opportunity when someone annoys me at work when I feel lonely, or fat or something. I want to plot against you.

I want to invent a potion for myself to drink every time I need you. Yes, I know, I summon you sometimes.

I hate you.

The black hole in some people makes them run while it makes others stop eating. Some people escape to books or something. You are demanding, and you want me to eat candy, for instance. And it's never enough. Or I'll buy things, and that won't be enough either.

A hole remains a hole.

I hate it when you're happy.

I hate you.

December 12, 2000

The score is 1:0 in my favor.

We haven't seen each other all day. Of course, it's a no-brainer because it's 1:00 a.m. and I've only just come back home, but still, I earned this point fairly. I didn't eat anything until 7 p.m. when I waited for Shai to come and eat with me. You dragged me to the deli to appease my hunger with some chocolate fluff cookie, but you lost, hole. I got off lightly, with a chewing gum, albeit with sugar, but still just chewing gum.

I feel very strong opposite you today, and maybe that's no biggie, but it's a small victory. Today you are weak.

I thought of giving you a name—maybe an imp, maybe not. An imp sounds like a term of endearment, and the best term of endearment I can give a black hole is a hole. Nothing more.

So dear hole, sleep on because I will sleep really well. I hope we won't see each other tomorrow, and if we do, I'll find a way to handle you. Today, I'm sure of it. I think I'm starting to recognize your weak spots and when you're extremely strong.

I noticed that in the company of some people, you're a real king. I noticed that when I wake up from an afternoon nap, you're extremely strong and that next to my folks you're the king of the world.

I think Mom is helping you without realizing it. Next to her, you're really sure of yourself. You almost always win. But this notion will help me shrink you, diminish your color until it's fully transparent. "Know thy enemy," the wise men said. And here I am, getting to know you.

I will eventually.

Wednesday, December 13, 2000

The score is 2:0 in my favor, hole.

I'm easily winning over you.

A full day. Your fault; you're the one weakening, and I'm prettier than ever.

I know the fact that I come home so late, toward bedtime, surely supports me, but I need a few more days like that in order to confront you face to face, you and I alone at home. Of course, the toughest battle of all is Friday evening at Mom and Dad's. That's your home field. Truly against all odds for me.

But anything can change. This slight feeling of victory from yesterday and today certainly fortifies me against you.

And today I am prettier than ever.

Friday, December 15, 2000

Hello, hole.

You almost won yesterday, but you didn't.

I saw you grow, I tried to shrink you with both hands, smash you, and you slipped between my fingers. I tried to smash you again, and you were like a monstrous playdoh, and you resisted. And you grew, and I fought you.

I was preparing a meal with Rony and Hagai. After the meal, I had a craving for something sweet. Rony handed me a candy bar, which I planned on sharing with her and Hagai. But they didn't want any, and you went into standby. You had ten minutes of bliss. It's okay. Mainly because later, and throughout the night, you called me, and I didn't respond, because I saw how black and miserable and mean you are. And I shrunk you. I know that today is testing day with you.

The real test.

Friday is always the hardest with you. But now it's 4 p.m., and I still haven't eaten. I hope I'll keep my sanity and remember you are ambushing me.

I hate you, hole, I gloat at your downfall.

I feel like I look great, and I'm not willing to give up this amazing feeling. I hope more than anything that I will win today.

Good-bye, hole, I hope we never meet again.

Friday, December 22, 2000

There was a boarding meeting on Wednesday.

The netherworld descended upon me a little, and you had a feast, hole.

You grew and puffed up and swelled up until you filled me entirely. You were no longer a hole, you were all of me. You occupied the entire space in my body. Everything a black, painful smoke, so that I couldn't even try to quiet you, exhale you out, or try to take control of you. I couldn't even talk to you, much less drive you away.

It's really scary. It's scary that I don't have the ability to stop for a moment because I know you the best, and I know it's your time, which is exactly why I need to get rid of you, not just when I'm strong and in control.

And I wanted to so badly, but I couldn't. I wanted to sit and write, but I guess I didn't really want to get rid of you because you were there and that's that.

I saw no point in talking to you because you had all the reasons to be there. And you didn't leave the next day, though I really wanted you to. I wanted to gain control over you once more and shrink you and be where I was the week before—strong and pretty and mainly in control.

I don't wish nor do I intend to suffer because of you, hole. Because of the birthday, I had two days of not very mindful eating, but not wild either. It was out of a decision to celebrate. Yesterday and the day before, you had the upper hand. And here's another place where you show up—always when I'm weak. And this time, it was the worthlessness and unkindness I felt toward myself, which really wasn't fair. You're the king of my weaknesses, hole.

You always glow when I feel bad.

Never mind that; it's your hostile takeover that I hate.

It's not that I think I always have to be in control. I want to train you to make me direct my anger or sadness to other places that aren't food, candy or anything else that attracts me to harm. I have to think of something.

Monday, December 25, 2000

I don't like you nor myself for that matter. Today I'm winning; I'm not losing to you. Not having much luck training you, but the fact that I can call you by name helps me. And sometimes, when you try to take over, I can still shrink you down to the size of a sweet. That's also something.

Today, for example, is a classic day for you to demand your "dough" because yesterday's discomfort was so great. A typical day for a donut and chocolate milk.

Still, the day somehow passed peacefully. Maybe it's no biggie, because I was very busy at work and maybe it wasn't fair to take the credit for a good day.

I feel you in my entire chest, trying to break the bars of my rib cage, pushing my heart to a corner, until it had not room to beat regularly. I know that here and now and today is the real test (one of many.)

I'm not fighting against your existence right now because I know there are good reasons for it. I'm only fighting the side effects of your existence.

I want you to leave, quietly, to evaporate, to dissipate, to vanish...

I feel that in this approach of mine (to vanish?!), I come off a little stronger perhaps. I don't wage war on you, but I'm also aware of your horrible side effects, which I'm not willing to accept. Don't add insult to injury. It's enough that I can't really breathe. And here we are busy negotiating. How funny. You're a terrorist seeking unlimited control over my body. And I'm a moderate diplomat, aiming for compromise. I acknowledge your existence, but I won't allow you to take over me. They will end up recruiting us for the peace negotiations.

Get lost, hole.

I'm waiting without losing my head.

***

You too, Tamar, see your black hole calling you, "Fill me up, stuff me, I can't stand this emptiness, this void inside me. I, too, wake up every time you weaken." And you try to fight it, fill it up.

In your own way.

I watch you curiously from the side, how you consciously, or perhaps unconsciously, choose the path you are on. Yesterday, for the first time since we embarked on our mutual journey, you wore slightly different clothes. Tighter, wrapping.

At the end of the session, when you turned to leave, I found myself imagining if and when you will be smaller. I thought to myself, you could look wonderful. You don't have a hiney and most of your fat it is in your stomach. You don't look so big from behind.

I wonder why the fat is in the front. It's more typical of male obesity. A round, apple-like fat. A belligerent, defiant fat.

Have you ever thought about it?

And what about the rest of the family members? How do they collaborate with or contribute to the existence and maintenance of this obesity?

Are they unconsciously preserving this huge, present, scary but so protective, warm and guarding place?

Nadav. Always there for you. As a holder? An accelerator? A container?

Last night, for the first time, you debated the nature of his function and presence. Up until now, we didn't talk much about him, your life partner. Only yesterday, he took an active part. And suddenly, you found out that you don't even know how this whole treatment resonates with him. What is he going through at the same time as you? Can it be that defying all reason, he is threatened by the treatment? Scared? And perhaps, unintentionally trying to sabotage it?

On Saturday night, he was the one who bought the huge popcorn box, who filled the fridge with tons of tempting rolls and bagels. Does his doing contain a non-verbal message or an expression of an unconscious conflict?

I shall go too far by asking if perhaps he is comfortable with your obesity. Just as your obesity serves you in protecting your promiscuous sexuality, the wantonness that you would otherwise be tempted to give in to, perhaps it protects Nadav? And could it be that your obesity leaves him comfortable, unthreatened, secure in his relationship, in the love, trust, and your assured existence in his life?

Nadav himself is busy with his own body, his excess weight and his recurring attempts to drop it. From that, he also shares the understanding and true loyalty to your hardship and inertia, since that is the story of his life.

The eating, cooking, and handling of food characterize your family. There is a connecting line between you that provides and fulfills, a sense of warmth, home, and giving. In Nadav's expert bread making, in your indulging Sushi cuisine, and mainly in containing and feeding. And you can't really give it up.

Because even your children are "marked" by the irresistible urge to eat, by truly taking pleasure in it, and by delighting in the special flavors of the dishes you and Nadav cook.

And your daughter, she looks so much like you. Tall, impressive, erect. With a strong tendency for overweight and a passionate love for food. She definitely appreciates a good meal. This scares you and drives you crazy, though you are careful not to intervene. Because how can you comment on it if you yourself are not a role model, and besides, who knows better than you how hard it is to practice restraint, to not give up?

And your son, too, is no different in his love of eating. Indeed, he is in the process of growing and is as thin as a rail, but you are anxious because you see the nature of eating and you realize what is fueling it. And that frightens you somewhat. Because just as you are anxious about yourself and find it hard to help yourself, you are twice as anxious about your kids.

We didn't go into it in depth. I think neither one of us was keen on touching on it nor finding out. And perhaps, we didn't really mean to get that deep.

December 24, 2000

You know, Tamar, something in me stopped. The enthusiasm of the start became a more realistic, contemplative, uncertain observation. It's not an easy process. It's far more complicated and intricate than I had imagined.

During the first years after I completed my studies, I believed I had the power to really make a difference, instigate changes, and lead people to better places with their bodies.

I truly believed that a suitable, mindful food plan was enough to lose weight. But bit by bit, I realized that most people find it hard to stick with weight loss frameworks. They tend to lose weight and then gain weight and so forth.

I began to realize that a written food plan and abiding by the dietician's rules was not enough. I recognized that in some cases, weight maintenance, albeit high, is better than the famous "yo-yo effect."

I learned that in order to help my patients, I have to be attentive to them, their needs and their abilities, which change at any given moment. And perhaps, because of that, Tamar, I was able to listen to you and understand what you were talking about when you spoke of your inner pace. Of the slow process you are undergoing, of the fear of exposure, of stripping. You were very preoccupied with how you gave yourself emotionally so quickly, how you surrendered almost entirely, so different from how you know yourself. And this surrender is different from your weight loss pace, which may be an accurate reflection of your familiar inner pace. And then, a discrepancy develops between your stronger emotional surrender and your ability to apply it and lose weight.

And the discrepancy has such a strong dissonance.

And what is my pace as a therapist?

Perhaps it's slower in me, too.

When we started the treatment, there was something delightful in it for me, and now, when the initial cloud of excitement has cleared, and we arrived at the hard, Sisyphean, nitty-gritty part, I got a little tired.

And here, I touch on the aspects that are complicated for me as a therapist.

In the world of eating disorders and obesity, there are many frustrating moments. Many times, I find myself busy with imparting strength, motivation, optimism. I often find myself trying not to sink into the indifference, despair, and helplessness of the patient. Since the hurdles are infinite, there is something very frustrating in the chronicity and the difficulty in experiencing real achievements.

And with you, Tamar, I sometimes feel like your dexterity in deep introspection is to your disadvantage and works against you. You're busy with emotional and cognitive insights and don't let yourself go with the process. Your preoccupation with why, with reasoning, sometimes reinforces the place you're stuck in and hinders you from acting.

Yes, I recognize small changes, but they aren't enough.

Your way of eating has changed, both in quantities and in the urge to eat. You eat more moderately, out of choice. There is something more temperate in your eating.

While your eating is still accompanied by much guilt and false beliefs that control it, you no longer engage in unconscious eating. You eat more mindfully. Something in effect associated with the eating has changed.

Tamar, if you succeed in acquiring tools that will enable you to see yourself through a less judgmental filter, perhaps your self-perception will change and allow you a more objective view of yourself. This can reinforce you.

And, in order to reinforce the change, let's become familiar with the thoughts that drive your eating. We will try to examine what stimulates these binges beyond thoughts and feelings. Because in essence, we both understand that these are rarely sensations of physiological hunger.

According to Agras, one can divide these triggers into three types:

External environment: includes the place and time in which the binge occurred. The type and quantities of food you choose to eat and the external factors in the environment that triggered the binge.

For you, Tamar, any external event serves as a reason. The smell of food in the nearby bakery, a stroll in the market on Friday with the smell of savory filo pastries mixed in with the look of colorful, tempting fruits and vegetables, or even just an ordinary visit to the neighborhood café. Any situation that brings you face to face with the aromas or sights of food arouses all your senses. You become alert, yearning, eager, and mostly unable to restrain yourself.

Social environment: includes the gamut of your interpersonal relationships.

Therefore, it is worth paying attention if you are alone or with friends during a binge. Who is next to you during such a binge and how would you describe your relationship with him? What was the nature and type of interaction that led to your binge? Was there an interpersonal conflict that affected you?

With you, it seems to me that interpersonal conflicts don't necessarily trigger binges. Unless they have implications that would make you withdraw into yourself and sink into your own self-judgment.

The internal environment: contains your thoughts, feelings, and inner hunger has much influence. And here, Tamar, I believe, lies most of your complexity, the nature of which we are trying to figure out.

I find that feelings of self-anger and frustration affect your eating tremendously. They dictate a pattern of self-punishment. For instance, your dissatisfaction from treating one of the children in the institution you work at; the fear of crossing the line between treatment and involvement in the child's life in a way that may confuse the relationship of therapist-child with that of mother-child. And then, you sit at night, obsessing over it, beating yourself until you bleed and eat.

December 26, 2000

Yesterday I celebrated forty-one years.

Nadav and I returned to places we had been two or three years ago, on my thirty-eighth birthday.

We went on a trip to Galilee.

We explored the area.

And I discovered the growths growing inside me, the sick cells that multiplied so fast.

And one day, erupted.

And one day, hurt.

And was already at the doctor's, who sent me for testing, and was hysterical, but not brave enough to say what she was afraid of.

And my hand pulled.

And I already knew.

I'd felt for a long time that cancer was nesting in me; I felt it talking to me on the inside, along the back. I felt the dull pain.

And I said, "I'm joking" to whomever I said it.

But I knew it was serious.

Only that week, when it became real, my defense mechanisms kicked in, and denial protected me. And I could enjoy the concert and the restaurant we went to on the trip.

And I didn't know my life was about to change forever.

And that it would never be the same as before the day we returned from up north.

Everything happened in these three years.

Everything and nothing.

I had another chance at life, and I chose it. And we did so much with it—Nadav, who discovered a whole wide world inside him, and I, too, yes I did, too.

And somehow, now, after three years, as I sit here before the white snowy Mt. Hermon, breathing the same air, in the same atmosphere, I see how we are letting it slide between our fingers, Nadav and I both.

It's a good time to reconnect with what I've found inside.

Nothing is obvious.

Find it again, Tamar, inside you. In islands of serenity and acceptance, forgiveness and love, which are inside you.

December 28, 2000

There was something sad about you, Tamar.

Touch me.

I didn't know where. How.

You were a different Tamar, one I didn't know.

You came with pain, with a load, authentic, without disguise.

At least with me, you allow yourself to be yourself, I thought.

Strange, in daily life, the deeper the pain and sorrow, the merrier you come off. The lower your emotional state is, the more intensely the environment experiences you. You're happy, joking, dressed colorfully and attractively, taking interest in others as if it were the most important thing to you. But it's all a pretense. Because what you really want to do is to lie around, stare into space, and maybe even feel sorry for yourself.

Again this gap.

Between your true self and the extroverted self—as with the body, as with the fat. Again this dissonance.

What would happen if you allowed your true feelings to be seen? If you allowed yourself to show what you really feel?

What things are hidden so deep inside you that you find so hard to reveal, see and show they exist?

I think it's all mixed up. You learned long ago that your mood fluctuates in waves, that there is not always a logical reason to explain its fluctuations. Sometimes, you are simply down, and this low can stick with you for weeks. And just as it comes, it goes. These are waves of light depression that don't hinder your functioning but weigh heavily on your soul.

I know that many times, your low mood is a result of disappointments and self-frustration. Perhaps by your method of working, the interpersonal relationship balance you blend into. At work, for instance, you try with all your might to lead the children you treat to create a change, whether by enlisting in the IDF or trying to wean themselves off drugs. I remember a child patient of yours, whose family began to disintegrate over the years, and you felt how the child was slipping, too. A little drugs, too many absences from school. And you decided to fight for him like only you know. You realized he was a talented artist, and that with the right kind of support and reinforcement, he could possibly be helped and rescued from deteriorating further. You helped him cultivate his hobbies; you fund-raised; you set up an impressive exhibition; and you paved his way to a more optimistic future. When it was time for him to be enlisted, and he was rejected, you fought for him to be enlisted. Together, you stood against all the possible frameworks until he was enlisted into the IDF's Raful Youth Project.[25] And then, when he was stationed in a different unit than what you expected, and you realized that the army would not help him develop in the areas important to him, you felt like you didn't fight enough or that you failed. And I remember you being angry at yourself, full of disappointment for not being able to help him all the way. And this anger and self-criticism hit you. For a moment, you forgot everything that you did and the amazing places he now reached. And you forgot that you really can't have it all and that it's wonderful the way it is. And then, the frustration paralyzed you, and you retreated into yourself, agonizing.

And the same goes for other areas. When you think you could have done more, you get angry with yourself. And, since you are so sensitive and attuned to every detail, you cannot move on and repress it. So then, every little event becomes intensified. Like a conflict with a work colleague, errors in your therapeutic judgment, over criticism of yourself, and examining your reactions under a magnifying glass.

Indeed, there are days when everything goes past you, but on other days, every little event becomes a hump.

The financial situation also affects you.

You work hard, as does Nadav, yet your bank account is caving under the burden of bills. You would be willing to accept it if you could only see options for a change, but the thought that this will always be the case depresses you, especially when you have so many desires, needs and fantasies. And then, the gap grows along with the frustration. This is another junction where you run into giving up, accepting.

And you said, "Ayelet, I can't believe I'm letting you see me in these points. That I'm letting to peek into my lowest points. Not trying to hide my gloomy mood. Letting you see it, feel it and even touch it. And to my surprise, I'm okay with it."

It was a strange session. A cloud of sadness, of depression, crawled over you. You were a little absentminded, unfocused. There wasn't a conversation or an explanatory, sharing talk. You couldn't.

You had a hard time with me sensing you, with not being able to hide.

But there was also something comfortable, relieving about it. You could be yourself, even for a bit. Tired. faded, and it was fine, for you and for me.

As for me?

What was I doing there?

I think I was sailing in my own world of melancholy.

Its depths enticing as always.

Deep inside, I connected and identified with you. I felt my own pain, laying sleepily, waiting to be touched. I didn't allow myself to stay there for too long. I knew very well how dangerous it was to be sucked into my own distress, which was inviting. Dangerous for me and especially for you, Tamar.

I gathered myself.

I went back to you, Tamar, feeling and being there for you. Softly, so as not to hurt, not to break apart, I tiptoed.

I just tried to contain and perhaps give some energy in the form of reinforcement.

I tried to connect with you on a tangible level of all things. I looked for points that would strengthen you in the most basic way possible. And, to my surprise, I found plenty. The way you in which you eat, the quantities that have gone down, the type of food you choose to eat.

Before, you would eat rich, fatty food without giving it much thought: pasta in Alfredo sauce, fried fish, yellow cheese and cakes. You would each whether it was tasty or not, worth spending the calories on or not. You would eat for the sake/ritual of eating, to fill up, to keep busy. You would eat anything from cooked food like lentils and rice and couscous to snacks like Fritos corn chips, popcorn, cakes, and desserts—indiscriminately.

And today? I see a different you, picking and choosing your foods, trying to assess their nutritional value, whether they are worth eating in terms of satiation, fullness, pleasure, and satisfaction.

You don't eat just for the sake of eating, but you enjoy and take pleasure in it.

You try to eat pasta in tomato sauce or olive oil, baked fish, and low-fat cheese. You insist on a variety of vegetables, raw and cooked, and eat little cereal.

I don't mean to illustrate a complete change, because these changes happen slowly, if at all. Still, the mindless eating is slowly making room for mindful eating with awareness and sometimes out of choice. This is different, less impulsive eating that is less compulsive.

I reflected it to you.
And you lost weight.
An entire kilogram.
And, for a moment, it seemed like you even liked it.

And this weight loss is different. It clearly demonstrates the process you are undergoing, Tamar. This slowness is different than the old ways of dieting, where you would drop a ton of kilograms very fast—15 Kgs. in a month. Perhaps it shows you the different place from which the current weight loss is happening.

Because this time, losing weight is a byproduct of accepting yourself.

I think something has happened to you to allow you to access your fat, feel it, talk to it, understand it. And perhaps, from that, also give it up (partially.) This losing weight is something internal, more connected. I think this acceptance can allow separation and maybe even surrender.

And this is what I believed was happening to you, Tamar.

Granted, there is no thunder and lightning or a major change in this process; it's a one-step-forward-two-steps-back kind of a process, a questioning, debating process happening at its own pace.

In your pace, Tamar. And perhaps, there lies its greatness.

There is a beginning.

An exploration. Discoveries.

And it might be easier to continue this way. No one is being disappointed, no one is being tested and there are no grades. The only measure is your inner experience as a person.

I think that is a lot.

January 8, 2001

It's been two weeks, and for the first time, I'm reading what I wrote last time.

And of course, got very frightened. It's not with Ayelet's; it's a different story. It's my life, but not here, not with Ayelet. It should come in a different journal.

So, most of it stayed inside, and some leaked out. And now, it's already two weeks later.

I'm starting to realize clearly, what I have known for a long time: my life is in waves. Sharp highs and lows of pain, limpness, and fatigue, versus a life full of vigor and interest. Alive and dead, changing every week, sometimes every day.

Life and death in strong intensities.

What's that got to do with my eating?

I still find it hard to identify inner factors that influence my eating, but there is a connection nonetheless.

When I let go of life and enter a state of defeat, with lots of sinking inward, I also let go of my struggle with food.

When I'm alive, less empty, with vigor, with plans, I manage to handle myself better with food.

Just as I told Ayelet, my natural state of eating is one that keeps me at my weight. It's a constant struggle for me to eat less; the effort it takes is unimaginable.

January 15, 2001

Hard. Like tearing.

Touching, not touching.

You tell me you are paying attention, that the eating is not only triggered by mood swings, but by the circumstances of life.

When life is understood and delineated, food is more ordered and regimented. The day is organized with clear plans of action, work hours, rising, and eating. There is breakfast, lunch and dinner, and occasional snacks.

But when life scatters, like on vacation, a trip abroad, or any event that deviates from the routine, you scatter along with it. And you love and know how to be scattered, Tamar. Because in your essence, you easily get sucked into many areas of interest, curious to discover and experience. And thus, food gets jumbled in response. And then, you can no longer be in charge of your eating, plan and be mindful. And, just like your agenda changes and goes out of whack, so does food.

You are capable of getting up in the morning and eating an omelet from two eggs, salad, and three slices of light bread; go to lunch at a restaurant, eat a rich dish of pasta with seafood followed by Pavlova with wild berries for dessert.

Then, when evening comes, and you're certain you will make do with a thin slice of watermelon. You're dragged to a café where you order a grilled cheese sandwich with ice-blended coffee. Luckily, you remembered to reduce the sugar and the iced-coffee. Twenty calories off the 2,700 you ate that day. And that's another day where you didn't binge. You only ate out of pleasure.

And when you describe food, I'm filled with guilt. Because your face lights up, glowing from the feelings of pleasure and longing, and who am I to spoil it for you by saying, "That's too much, you could have at least given up the Pavlova and not eaten an omelet for breakfast?"

And this is only one example. Because some days can be a lot heavier, with not just three meals, but one ongoing meal the entire day, with no hunger point, no order, no awareness. The day could start with two sandwiches with light bread, then as you cook in the kitchen, you taste all the ingredients and then final products, the quiches, salads, and fish. And the tasting spoon is a teaspoon. Just the tasting comes out to about 1,000 calories, which you never felt or remembered you ate. Then it's lunchtime, and like everyone else, you sit down to eat. After all, you hadn't eaten anything since breakfast. And, in the afternoon, it's coffee with a small piece of cake, dry but nonetheless...

And, in the evening, you're invited to a bar mitzvah, and though you're filled with self-loathing, everything is tempting and tasty there. And you cannot resist it. And you forget to think and try to choose, and eat from everything. As if you haven't already wasted close to 2,500 calories.

Your scattering tendency, as I said, can be in all areas. Because everything is tempting and alluring. It's hard for you to give up something and feel disappointed. And the same goes for men. This flirting, the ability to conquer, tease, make your body quiver; you find it hard not to respond to them.

And then, you summon boundaries to you, to close off and block you in places where you can't do it. And you run wild only in those boundaries you have set for yourself.

You work in a job with clear rules and defined hours, but you work with delinquent, problematic, rule-bending and challenging youth.

The daily life in the institution you run is exhilarating, shocking and unpredictable. Constantly within the boundaries and outside them.

The same with me; you feel like you belong to our framework, you try to show up for the sessions, but in them, there are constant deviations and changes. No week is the same as the previous one. And there is never a guarantee that you will show up on time or at all. The most important thing is that there is a framework, but you make your own rules within it.

You say you noticed that it's easier for you to lose weight in the winter than in the summer. You feel better about yourself. In winter you don't sweat, you're less heavy and cumbersome. There are clothes that cover up and hide, not showing everybody your disgrace, your fat, your size.

But it's not just that. Losing weight in winter is less intimidating. You don't see, you don't know; it's all hidden. And then, you're not exposed, and you're not afraid of that thinner place. Because when everyone compliments you and pays attention, you immediately get anxious and ruin things.

What is amazing is that you've been calling attention to yourself all this time, but in different ways. You're always dressed intriguingly, colorful, unique. I noticed you like white and turquoise—that you invest a lot in shoes, mostly bulky, and in various colors. Somehow, you're always at the center of attention. There isn't a social situation that would find you in the shadow, in a corner. With your typical wit, you make your way back to center stage, where you bloom, full of adrenaline.

So what is in these compliments about your good looks and how you must have lost some weight that frightens you so? Perhaps what intimidates you is not the attention, which you are used to, but the focus on your body and on the weight loss.

We held a conversation that crossed lines. Boundaries?
We switched hats.
You mirrored me to myself. The reclusiveness. You wondered aloud about my being a person protective of her privacy. You spoke about the way I sit. Like a snail, you said, snuggled within himself. And, just like the snail, fragile to the touch.
And for a moment, I let you speak, I got carried away elsewhere, and I liked it. I liked not having to lead or guide. I liked being in a place where I was talked about. I was examined, asked. You spoke, and I listened.

You mainly spoke about the difference between the Ayelet inside the clinic and Ayelet outside of it. The Ayelet that brings herself to the therapeutic session ready and willing to be somewhat open and exposed, because here she is protected, and if someone frightens or touches her too much, she can immediately hide behind the figure of the distant, boundary-keeping therapist.

You spoke about my ability to give of myself only in areas where there was no real fear of being genuinely exposed—areas where I manage and control. Whereas outside, everything locks hermetically. No one leaves, and surely no one enters. The gap is huge, and the distance even further.

I asked myself if I allowed you to gain access because I trusted you, or because I was too tried to guard myself. And maybe I enjoyed it.

And you, with all your size, gently accessed.

You hesitated; how far? And I allowed it and liked it.

Not too deep, and surely not piercing, but accessing.

I suppose that deep down in my soul, I like being the patient sometimes. It facilitates a place of weakness, or helplessness, which I sometimes like to be in.

Sometimes; not a lot.

To feel it, to know what happens there, and then, mak a choice based on experience, on knowing, to go back to the strong, controlling, knowing and leading position. Only then, return to the place I am always at as a therapist and a person.

I felt that it didn't hinder the treatment, it was allowed. I'm not sure if it was really so.

Is it okay to let go every once in a while and enable the boundary between the therapist and the patient to be less rigid? And, if it can benefit the patient, is it legitimate?

Tamar, I felt that it allowed you to be in a position of power for a few minutes, a giving rather than a receiving place. There is something in the feeling of equality that creates closeness and connects. There is no therapist-patient temporarily, but a shift in the hierarchy, a different distribution of power.

And perhaps, that is a different experience.

What do I notice when a patient walks in for the first time?

I think it's the eyes. I examine their expression, their language.

Shira's eyes cried silently.

A deep blue, slightly slanted. The dampness, as if refusing to disappear, perpetuating the fatigue of a young woman in the spring of her life and the height of her misery.

The influx of words was gushed. It's as if she had accumulated a horde of emotions just waiting to for their time to ooze.

Shira. Soft, fair hair, gently cascading on broad shoulders. Tall, refined.

I watched her, examining every part of her long, slightly hunched body. Tight jeans, a blouse revealing a little of her belly; low cleavage emphasizing her femininity; and fashionable high heels with a matching purse—twenty-one years old; released from the army.

Surrounded by a loving family, guy friends, girlfriends. At the onset of her adult life, at the end of one stage and the beginning of another. But in fact, she didn't even exist. She was turned off, sunken, biding time and mainly confused, it seemed to me.

She said she came to lose weight.

I wondered what brought Shira to sit opposite me, and out of genuine distress, talk about her strong desire to drop 3 Kgs—as if her entire world depended on it.

There was a huge muddle of burning pain that can be summed up in one word—food. A battle with food, an endless war, where there were no winners or losers.

From the moment food invaded Shira's life, it didn't stop tricking her.

What role did it have? Why did Shira, who looked wonderful, need it?

Maybe when she understood that food is not an entity, but only a means—and that she must shift her preoccupation with the nerve-wracking struggle with food to understanding herself—she would be able to move forward.

She walked in overwhelmed. And from the moment she sat in front of me, it were as if a huge floodgate opened and the water came cascading down.

Shira, so I realized, built an entire life story around her body and the binges she developed. There was something naïve, inviting about her that didn't quite understand the attack that raged on her life. But sadness had already settled in. Suffering and pain dwelled safely inside her, warming up their bones, as if knowing they were on safe ground.

She was still hung up on weight as a number. She was at three kilos.

How could I break the news to her that the treatment is more complex?

That it's not just three kilos, but perhaps a mixture of emotions.

I asked myself how she would feel better with her inner world, which is actually guarding those three kilos and binges adamantly, refusing to part with them.

Her inner world takes care of it, cushions it. Does anything but touch it, but understand it, but uncover its true needs and wishes.

And what are three kilos?

Two weeks of dieting and they're gone.

Two weeks of 1,000 calories with a structured, ordered plan and she is "thin."

Just keep your mouth closed, and they're gone.

But maybe these three Kgs. are something much greater than three Kgs.?

Shira.

A normal home, a warm, close family, life on a normal track without any dramatic life events.

And an enemy.

From our first meeting, I found out that she had been to a psychological treatment that was cut short due to her guilt about wasting her parents' money, as well as her immaturity to cope and work on herself.

I think Shira's difficulty stemmed from her high self-critique, from an idealist perception of reality, and an intensification of every feeling. Thus, she found it hard to accept and to cope.

Because everything was so vulnerable and exposed.

So, instead of touching that painful and confusing emotion, she was preoccupied with food. There, it seems, things were far simpler: you eat to feel and not to feel; you eat to not know, not exist.

And then, it's seemingly easier, legitimate, and practical.

Shira is completely preoccupied with her appearance and the three extra Kgs. But, aside from the weight, she is terrified from the binges and her inability to control food. These binges can show up even several times a day. So, when she returns home, and the house is empty, she can eat two bars of chocolate, a bag of savory pretzels dipped in white cheese, and a generous helping of ice cream. That amounts to nearly three thousand calories.

Left helpless after the binge, lethargic by the food and the terrible thoughts about being weak and spineless, she shut herself in her room, crying, lamenting her behavior and her weight gain. She detached from her girlfriends and parents and was busy being angry at herself and her horrible behavior. This type of incident can repeat itself, each time with a different outcome. For instance, if she goes out with a guy, and she feels uncomfortable with him or disappointed that he doesn't fancy her, she will come home and fill herself up on a few slices of bread with a spread, ten chocolate truffles and a large bowl of cereal with milk. Then the usual ritual: locking herself in the room, cutting off any communication with the environment, and hiding under the blanket; and this depression could last hours or even whole days. In this state, she hardly eats.

Shira lives in constant fear of the next binge, if she will be able to control it or will it take over her. She feels it lurking in every corner. She doesn't always know what it wants from her and when it will erupt, what its intensity will be and how long it will make her life miserable. But she knows it's coming.

Because almost any emotional jolt summons it to invade her.

But it will come when it feels like it; no prior notice or consultation.

So, she waits.

In the therapeutic process, Shira tried to understand the nature of these binges. What triggers them and what postpones them? She realized she needed them to shift the intensity of her emotions, which she found hard to contain. She began to see that emotionally charged situations created disquiet and a dull pain in her, prompting a binge, followed by a period of barely eating. Thus, she found herself living from one binge to the next.

Three months have gone by. Shira is in a different place.

She works, has a boyfriend; still at the same weight, but in a different place.

Her mood swings subsided, and her relationship with her weight and body has taken a different turn. She has learned to accept herself and love herself a little more.

And it's not that she is pleased with her body weight or appearance, but she has learned to live beside it with small compromises that enable her to enjoy life and function daily without falling into the depths of her inviting bed or hiding behind endless tears and internal quarantine orders.

But there is still a cloud hanging over her, threatening every now and then to taint her soul. And sometimes, it's enough that she ate a bar of chocolate the day before, or any type of food she deems forbidden, to paint her entire world a somber black.

And don't get me wrong, she looks amazing.

But it's as if something in her still finds it hard to give up the pain.

Shira has made huge leaps.

Her binges have minimized. They are more internal than real. In actuality, if she eats a bar of chocolate, it's not followed by a bag of peanuts, ice cream, and other high-calorie snacks. She is able to make do with chocolate as dinner.

She doesn't eat many calories.

But she is still possessed by irrational beliefs and thoughts regarding certain foods she eats. That is, the very consumption of these foods, which she perceives are unhealthy and fattening, can trigger a binge.

So for example, if she ate a slice of pizza or a hamburger, in her mind, she ate a forbidden food the very consumption of which could ruin her diet, her existence as a controlled person, dragging her once more into major binges.

This behavior confuses her, causes her major guilt, pain, and suffering, even if this eating doesn't lead to weight gain.

These situations quickly catapult her into an experience of helplessness and low self-esteem. Not only does she belittle herself and feel bad about her appearance, but she also projects her feelings onto those surrounding her. As if they see and know her powerlessness.

When we look at her change, we discover that the depression no longer consumes her, runs her life, or keeps her locked up at home. But it's still there. It still knocks on her door every now and then, threatening to undermine her confidence and self-love.

Shira.

Her eyes are gleaming, and at times, it seems like she doesn't rest for a moment. Her mind is constantly working, thinking for herself, for others, exhausting, nagging thoughts, going in circles and not letting her escape. Some pertain to food and weight:

- Can't eat anything high-caloric because touching it, even a little, will make me fat."
- "If I don't lose those three kilograms, I won't be happy."
- "I'm weak, unworthy, with no will power."
- "I must never eat chocolate."

Some of those thoughts center on her interpersonal relationships, revealing strong judgment and criticism of herself.

And letting them go is not easy.

Is she even capable of giving them up?

And what do I mean by that?

Shira is holding onto the obsession with food as an anchor and a guarantee that she would not really gain weight. Because what would happen if she let go of the pain and suffering for a moment?

What would happen if she ate a bar of chocolate and didn't feel guilty about it?

What would happen if, after such eating, she wouldn't torment her body and soul and beat herself up?

In her perception, if she let go and ate those forbidden foods without being punished, she would open the door to more binges, followed by weight gain. Because if she opened the door just a crack, how could she guarantee that the crack wouldn't expand and break down the boundaries?

Especially when Shira's list of forbidden foods is so long: pasta, pizza, crackers, chocolate, ice cream, jam, French fries, pita, whole milk, sweets, cream and whipped cream, cookies and cereal. How can you live life with so many prohibitions without deviation?

Is it possible that the anxiety and fear of the what if sustains the obsession?

At the end of the session, Shira smiles— somewhat to herself, and somewhat to me.

Self-conscious and perhaps embarrassed.

I already said she looks amazing. And where does it say that one needs to be "thin" in order to look and mainly feel amazing?

And Shira knows it intellectually, but she is still in the process of internalizing it.

She understands it logically, but she still can't run her life accordingly. Only partially.

Perhaps this is our next therapeutic destination.

Six months later.

I felt it was time for an interim assessment of the treatment. She had a hard time seeing where she had started.

"Did I really feel that way?" she asked. "Was I really in such a low place? Did the food put me in such painful places that I wasn't there for myself, my family and my friends?"

She shed a tear.

She felt sad about the places she had been to and the difficulty she experienced. The pain.

She looked back and knew. She was no longer there; she was completely elsewhere.

Not thinner, but it doesn't affect her happiness or social connections.

Not thinner, but food no longer runs her life.

Recognizing her worth, skills and abilities, which are not dependent on what and how much she ate; she even weighed herself and wasn't startled by the fact that the weight didn't change.

Because what does it matter? The most important thing is that she is happy, she looks and feels wonderful, and she knows it.

Yesterday, she shared with me the ending of a short, but meaningful relationship. She was sad for it; she felt the pain of separation. But she didn't direct it to the food. She spoke of the pain, felt it, knew it.

She didn't entrench herself in binges or stock up on candy. She did touch chocolate, but not as a remedy for the soul.

I felt her.

And her smiling eyes gave me pleasure.

January 22, 2001

One minute, I'm convinced we will succeed, and the next, I wonder. Hesitant.

I knew it would be hard, long; I didn't know just how much.

I knew it was important to you, and to me, that something would happen as a result of the treatment. Something that hasn't happened yet. But the change was late to come.

I feel the pain and frustration pent up inside you, your inability to watch, to reduce the quantities significantly, and mainly your inability to create this change that would result in weight loss. Should you give up the journey? Deep down you know you shouldn't, that you mustn't. Giving up for you means worsening. From your experience, when you give up and choose not to be aware of your eating, your weight skyrockets. You also know and feel what those many kilograms mean for you: a raging blood pressure, a sugar value of 168 and a lot of physical discomfort. What's said is that the more intensified and intimidating the kilograms become, the weaker and more fatigued you become. The journey seems longer and impossible.

Tamar, I know you mustn't give up because agreeing to this size and fat is also agreeing to ailment and heaviness. I want to clarify myself. I'm not pulling you toward being thin, but toward losing weight in a way that would make you feel healthier and lighter.

Ten to fifteen percent of your current weight.
About 15 Kgs.

And just as Hila writes:

I opened the closet door to find something to wear to work tomorrow, But 80 percent of my beautiful clothes don't fit me. I have almost twelve pairs of pants. Each one nicer than the other. Jeans, black pants, greenish pants, maroon, blue, plaid-blue…such a shame.
I hardly have anything to wear now.
I'm starting Herbalife tomorrow.
I'm starting a diet tomorrow.
I don't really feel like analyzing the situation. It's hard. It's hard to stand, to get out of bed, to wipe my butt, to walk a lot. I'm uncomfortable with my belly.
I feel like I'm starting a rehab/detox program.
Drug rehabilitation.

Tamar, your ability to give up large quantities of food is also perceived at times as a detox process—detoxifying from food and the rituals that come with it.
But unlike drugs, without which our body can physically exist, we cannot survive without food. We cannot detach

from it completely. Therefore, a complete detox isn't possible. We have to learn to walk that fine line between a little and a lot, between with and without. In fact, the hardest thing for us to learn is how to stay in the middle. Extremes are easier, whether it be huge quantities or near-fasting. The challenge is in finding the balance.

I believe that balanced eating isn't achieved through the extremities. On the contrary, they are what makes finding the middle ground difficult. Yet, this time, I considered trying to offer you a "project." I thought it might help spark that fire in you and infuse you with vitality and a desire to fight for yourself. I thought that an immediate loss of a few kilograms would spur the joy of effort in you. For that purpose, I recruited the antibiotic in my possession, which I so hate to use, and told you that maybe if we tried a "starvation diet" to drop off two to three kilograms immediately, it might temporarily arouse the motivation that would set the ball rolling and ignite the energy deposits depleted in you.

To do that, we decided that you would follow a written plan for a week.

I wonder where this will experience will take us. We both realize that the problem isn't physical. If you watch it, you'll lose. If you watch it, the kilograms will fly off. But there is a catch to it. There is something very tempting in an instant solution like that. As if some kind of magic solves the problems. You just keep your mouth shut for a little bit, and you lose weight. A breeze.

And perhaps, this is where the main problem lays—the term "diet" and what it may provoke in us.

There are a few types of diets:

1. Abstinence: People who try to abstain from eating for as long as possible, sometimes until the evening hours, or alternately, try to reduce the amount of times they eat per day.
2. Limitation of caloric intake: The attempt to ensure food consumption below a certain number of calories. The caloric reduction may even reach 600–800 calories per day.
3. Reducing or limiting certain types of food or food groups (pizza, cookies, sugars): Thinking that certain foods are forbidden and eating them will lead to weight gain or binges. Therefore, they are divided into "allowed" and "forbidden." Researchers have shown that one of five women of the entire population controls her eating in this way.
4. Creating structured, dictated eating plans that will influence body shape and weight: That is, relying on a few external rules to tell us when, how much, what or not to eat. This is the classic diet.[26]

Many times, abstinence arouses feelings of deprivation, guilt, and self-contempt. These trigger binges and loss of control over eating (the abstinence theories mentioned in the foreword.) Each one of these ways represents a method that monitors and tries to control a person's eating. It gives him

---

[26]Christopher G. Fairburn, *Overcoming Binge Eating*. The Guilford Press, 1995.

external boundaries for eating, but doesn't really develop his inner boundaries and listen to his true needs, his inner hunger.

I was wondering whether to risk providing a structured, dictated plan as a motivation initiator, while realizing it may trigger a binge.

I shared it with you.

We pondered it and weighed the pros here and there and realized that the place you are in, which was low anyway, we had to give it a try.

I felt your fear, your hesitation.

"What if I won't be able to follow the instructions and do exactly as you wrote," you said. "And besides, you realize I haven't dieted in a long time or eaten according to a plan. I know I'm stuck and unable to pull myself together for our journey, but who can guarantee I'll pull myself together for this one? What if I don't? Will I add another failure to my name? Another disappointment?"

"You're right," I answered, "but if we don't try, we won't know, and as it is, you're not moving in any direction. You're stuck. So maybe this attempt will advance you and create a beginning."

We decided to gamble on it.

We agreed on a food plan that included:

- Twelve slices of light bread
- One container of 5 percent cheese

- Vegetables of all kinds, cooked and fresh, without limitation
- Two pieces of fruit
- Two cups of coffee

Only a week, we said.

January 30, 2001

I haven't done it in so many years.

I haven't practiced it.

I haven't dealt with it.

I already said that my preoccupation and connection to myself regarding the obesity is part of my heavy, depressed mood lately.

I usually somehow live separate from the awareness that I'm so fat, that I'm so abnormal with food. Because within this pathology, I live "normally" with awareness and heavy feelings on the one hand, but a lot of indecision on the other. I radiate a lot of confidence and power to my environment. It happens when I forget I'm so huge and when I'm living my less physical being.

During such times, all of my other dualities come out, and I'm not preoccupied with being fat.

Then I manage to be active, energetic, attractive, funny.

When I connect to my fat self, I get pulled down—to heaviness, to depression.

In my treatment with Ayelet, I was asked to maintain my fat awareness all the time in order to confront it, and that's hard.

Ayelet.

Lately, I haven't written at all. I'm more reclusive, less allowing, less touching.

I'm getting to know Ayelet little by little although she is introverted.

It's not easy. Because if she were only a therapist, she would interest me just that much. And then, it's superficial and simple. But, as always, nothing is simple.

I'm learning about her, her taste, her demands of herself, her values, her pace, and lifestyle.

Just a little.

We are different, like water and stone.

And she is foreign to me and at the same time not.

She is so different from me.

She brings herself as an understatement, closed up, occupying little space.

And me—with all my size and wild presence.

Although her quiet intensity peeks and is seen by those who look carefully.

I understand my attraction to her now, when she allows herself to be in the poems. In addition, there, I can connect to this well. And from there, I understand my source of interest in her. Because it stems from a place that is close to me.

Her wonderful poetry brings her closer to me.

And her shield—deters me.

I'm also dissuaded by her interest in my life and the fact that through food, she inspects my life. Where I was and with whom. Because when we review the week through food, it's my way of life.

And, all of a sudden, she knows what I'm doing and when, and what Nadav is doing. This voyeurism is hard for me and deters me. Distances me. This familiarity with my life is difficult and shuts me down, taking away my privacy.

I need this discreetness and privacy of not letting anybody in.

Ayelet also finds it hard if we talk about her, her life, her pain and joy. Sometimes, she allows it a little but immediately backs off.

It's a little confusing.

Because in this treatment, I'm the patient and she's the therapist, and she makes sure not to bring herself personally into it.

And I find her interesting.

Because, sometimes, we touch each other's lives even outside this reality.

And I ask myself, if through reviewing what you eat and when, Ayelet is satisfying some voyeuristic need of hers to invade her patients' lives, as I have satisfied and still do, my own voyeuristic need of invading the lives of the children I treat.

And I know there is no other way. This report on food is right for me, but it's also daunting for me. This is probably why I needed to distance myself a little.

I look at how she holds herself. Gathered, contracted all the time.

In her body language, too, mainly in her lips.

And I wonder where you get the strength to hold yourself with such stress all the time. With such constant control, such precise planning, and the need to have it all your way.

Through the wall.

Domineering life.

In a constant, precise super-plan that takes her to all the places she wishes to get to. At least we have her poems. This for me is the main point of connection. Because this is where everything hides behind that starched curtain.

I have let go big time in the last one to two months. I was overtaken by a terrible mood. Lack of will, inability, indifference or everything together. The excitement of the beginning waned. I started to get bored by the routine. I ate a lot less than before, but not in order to lose weight.

I agree with Ayelet that I eat with more control and less impulsiveness, but not in order to lose weight. And in the last weeks, mainly weekends, I gorged. And then, during the week I would lose it, then gain it back over the weekend. And this is a familiar story carried over from old diets.

We were both stuck. Ayelet with her will to conquer the mountain, and me, powerless, sad, defeated, but not entirely. Like I told Ayelet, there is still some basic desire in me to take up that one-time glove which was thrown at me.

And then, within this dreariness and desperation, Ayelet with her vigor and strength, took it another step forward. To another week. A little more extreme. And suddenly, I was able to gather myself and gain power.

I'm in a better mood, with more strength so I can do.

I did, and I lost, and I came happily with strength to carry on and an ability to eat less, give up, say no and postpone gratification. We'll see how the weekend goes. And mainly, a Saturday with Meir, whose workshop I'm hosting at my house.

We'll see how long this whole thing lasts.

Ayelet ran into my little "manic-depressions" I have been experiencing in the last few years.

This time, the "blues" around my birthday were really physically painful, and I couldn't pick myself up. It took over a month. And now, I'm in a good period, not free of relapses, but small ones. I remember that as a kid reading children's books, I was most stimulated by what they ate. And I remember those parts very well. Later, when I would eat, I would imagine myself inside the story and derive great pleasure from it.

For instance, in the book Sophie's Misfortunes by Countess of Ségur.

All the girls there were pretty, slender, charming and possessing great manners. Only Sophie, a distant cousin, was round and sloppy and of course, most of all, naughty and full of mischief.

One time, she escapes and reaches the windmill where the bread is baked. She steals a loaf of fresh, dark bread with crunchy crust that smells amazing, and swipes fresh crème off the windmill's pantry. Then, sitting hidden, she breaks the oily cream crust with the fresh bread and lifts the bunch to her mouth.

She consumes an entire loaf with a full jar of cream.

Naturally, her punishment isn't late to come as she writes with stomach pain due to her huge binge.

Since it is a known fact that one mustn't eat fresh bread straight from the oven. Especially when it's stolen. I read that tantalizing description at least a hundred times.

I was maybe eight years old.

And the same as an adult. I remember places abroad by what we ate, where and when. Of course, there are other experiences that activate other senses, the second after taste being touch. The physical contact with skin, air, water, wall, earth. And only then, through smell and then sight.

Totally out of whack.

Normal people first see, then comes all the rest.

Touch for me is mainly in the hands and face, and mostly fluid, rough things, and smells.

I think that my glasses, not just the fat, protect me from the intense world I have stumbled upon with extra hyper-sensitivity.

I hear too well, and I hear everything.

At work, I am available to three or four people and a few events simultaneously. I can't respond to them all, but I hear everything, even when I'm focused on just one, and people are boggled by how I can respond concurrently, even to the psychopaths, the sick and the listless arriving on the first day.

The world is too cramped and it's hard to shrink the aperture, thicken the filters, and this fat is an insulating Styrofoam layer, and why get rid of it really? It's like Meir Shalev's[27] story about the kid who chose to look at the world without glasses so as not to see too clearly.

So why choose differently?

It's so comforting, I'm so used to it.

And it's such a great effort to connect.

Aside from health, all the other benefits are dangerous and intimidating. Who said I could allow myself to look good?

Who said I could look normal?

Maybe I can't even deal with it.

As it is, I'm so flighty, what will happen if I'm actually light?

The fear of dying is certainly a good reason that motivates me, and the desire to gain a better quality of life, to enjoy life more. After all, I'm a glutton.

And I want to enjoy as much as I can.

But I also want to sink, or I let myself sink.

I get a fright when my sugar or blood pressure skyrockets, but only for a short period.

It motivates me to lose a kilo or two, and that's it.

I'm not truly able to be responsible for my health, and think about my young children; after all, I want to be their mother for many years to come.

I thought that after I touched death when I got sick, I would take more responsibility for my health. So, it was like that for the first year or two after the treatments, then slowly but surely it faded. Meir says that a good fear is one that turns into an

---

[27] An Israeli writer and a publicist.

urge. So, *my fear of death turned into an urge. It dissolved. And I didn't really take my chance for a healthier life.*

Stay with your desire to be healthy for a little.
Keep that vigor for another few weeks, Tamar, before the next dipping; lose about ten kilograms before you sink again. And then, rest…rest…
And Ayelet, who constantly needs to move mountains, will move slowly with me, and that is her lesson.

February 5, 2001

So, you accepted the challenge, Tamar. And you even lost some weight.

It wasn't easy for you, but nonetheless, you made an effort.

Sure, it wasn't exactly according to plan and with many deviations. But all in all, you were in it. You kept the general structure or twelve slices of light bread, Quark cheese and vegetables.

Can you really stick to a structured plan? How can a person know what he would like to eat in advance at a certain moment or hour? And you, of all people, full of surprises, needs, and urges.

So, within this rigid food plan, you found your little emergency exits that enabled you to be present most of the time and a little absent.

Every day, you garnished the "menu" differently.

One time, you ate a fish for lunch, another time you added a few cookies, but only a few. And there was one day when you took it one step further and chose to only eat a large, fulfilling lunch at a restaurant and made do with fruit for dinner. And it was all good, since, within the chaos, there was suddenly some order and some surrendering.

And, as said, you lost weight. Not a lot, but you did.

1.100 Kgs. (2.42 Lbs.)

February 15, 2001

The second session of reading to each other what we had written over time was difficult. There was something else that wasn't there in the first session—heaviness; sadness.

We didn't look into each other's eyes; they were tearful.

We couldn't speak; the words refused to be uttered.

At least we had the poems, which we wrote. They broke the silence.

So we read.

Ayelet:
> In butterflies of sapphire
> You buried
> Specks of tears
> You followed the sound of
> Silence
> As a naked bride wears
> A winter veil.
> Butterflies unraveled your
> Torso
> Your estrangement watched you
> Change.

Tamar:

As if you weren't
Kicking your legs
As if you weren't
Holding onto liquid sand
That knows how to betray.

Ayelet:

His breath
Swallowed the residues of
Her bubble
Biting delicately
Her wounds
Burning
Smelling of Wormwood.

Tamar:

Silver foil
Wrapping shattered lungs
Gushing nectar
To
The pores of the tongue.

Ayelet:

Fall
Unripe leaves
Drew a wary tongue
The lust flooded furrowed
Clods

Unripe leaves paved burning leaf tears
Grabbing humiliated thighs

Tomorrow's clouds stretched
A gray blanket
Snuggled in yesterday's drought.

Tamar:
We tied long ribbons that fluttered
In the peninsula's heat wave.

We descended into steaming swamps
Of desire

There we met the cold spout
Gleaming
Inside a rocking hammock.

Endless exhales
Peeled the thick skin
Of what was left.

Evil
Evil crawls under
The smile of a tiny, dark tree

I have forgiven the stones on the road
I have forgiven the curb
That carried us
So heavy
Because only then were we born.

You read.

I read.

The lines carried on a conversation, a strange dialogue.

There was a lot of intimacy in the room. Airless. We felt each other.

I felt your despair and helplessness in the battle against the fat and against yourself. You felt my despair and helplessness at the stagnancy, your inability to fight for yourself.

And in the room, our feelings blended with your tears, gently appearing and clouding the lenses of your glasses with salty clouds of mist.

And that fat.

Separating us.

And you hurting, your illnesses destroying every organ in your body. The ups and downs wreaking havoc in your soul. And your huge, awkward body, binding and slashing you.

I couldn't look up.

> Layers of dust that weathered the weights of her body
> A silent memorial.
> A blubbery life buoy,
> Wrapping it, sinking down the blackened abyss.
> Sheep droppings lining golden lairs,
> Afraid to glimpse
> Or else they will be corroded at once.

February 16, 2001

Our meeting was almost unbearable. We read what we wrote, poems, too, and that's it.

Suddenly, we could hardly say a thing to each other.

It was so painful.

What's the point of all these words? You always end up with the pain. They don't ease anything.

Ayelet hardly dared to look at me, or I at her. Each one buried our eyes in the words, and I found no salvation, no ease, or comfort in them.

No comfort.

Ultimately, it's you with yourself, the heaviness, the mountains of fat, the explanations, interpretations, the words poured on top don't change what's underneath.

Perhaps the words, like food, are a false attempt to hide the pain. Food enters and the words pour out.

I'm not really able to break out of this,

I'm stuck in this trap, and everything I rely on is false.

I feel like taking off.

March 1, 2001

Strange, for some time now, I haven't felt the need or ability to write.

I wonder.

Perhaps I'm mad. At you. At myself.

Perhaps disappointed. With you. With myself.

I was hoping you would come to the session; that we could talk, understand.

That you cope with the stagnancy, the binges, the disappointments.

But you chose to continue hiding.

From yourself.

From me.

March 22, 2001

I failed again.

March 26, 2001

After weeks during which I couldn't write, I found a way that would connect me to you differently, through a poem by Adam Zagajewski:[28]

How does the man look who's right
What kind of tie does he wear
Does he speak in complete sentences
Does he dress in well-worn clothes
Did he walk out of a sea of blood or
A sea of oblivion do his clothes still
Bear traces of sharp-tasting salt
What era is this man from
Is his skin sallow
Does he cry in his sleep what does he dream of
Always the same room
With the wall's extracted heart does he talk
To himself does he live in an old man's
Rented body how much unrest
Does this cubicle cost him is he an exile

---

[28] A Polish poet, novelist, translator, and essayist. The poem is published in his collection *Without End*. Farrar, Straus & Giroux, New York, 2002.

From what city is it curiosity
That drives him is it worth it
Who answers for this what's that stain
On his coat who stands behind him
Could you tell him that everything is
Relative depending on how you look at it
No one knows how it really is
See if you can recognize him
As he crosses the street
Hunched beneath the weight of brains.

What is motivating you, Tamar?

Is it worthwhile?

Do you always hide in that same room when you run away from me, from yourself?

Does it feel like you're in exile from yourself, disconnected from feeling?

And besides, what does it feel like to be exiled from yourself?

Or do you not feel anything whatsoever, and that's what it's all about.

What is that space you have gotten yourself into?

Is it big?

Does it have windows?

Or maybe it's sealed?

Empty?

And then, after running away and disconnecting from yourself and from me, do you still believe I can recognize you when you walk down the street hunched over by the burden of your body, the burden of your life? What else do you need to experience in order to reach a place where you stop wandering and are able to break free from your chains?

"Aye," you said, "you're touching me in the most painful places. I wish I knew what to answer you. After all, I've been meddling in these places for years. Asking myself and finding it hard to answer. When you pose these questions so directly and blatantly, do you think I'd have an answer? I wish I'd understand my choices; my disconnection through food; my hiding in the coffin I built around my body."

I tried to see your withdrawal into that narrow, crowded space you escaped to from yourself. But despite my understanding, I think I was mad, disappointed. And perhaps, you because you took time off, I did too.

How did I dare? After all, it was my job to keep guard.

But can I be responsible for something I am not responsible for? Can I care for someone who doesn't care for himself? I'm not prepared to assume responsibility for what is beyond my control. I'm not prepared to feel guilty by someone's failure. Did I allude to that? Did I, as usual, do it without words?

After all, I invited you on the journey, gave you a backpack with excellent gear, a perfectly drawn out map, a guide who knows every nook and cranny. I knew what was ahead of you, and I tried with all my heart to steer you in the right direction. But you perhaps listened and perhaps not, you chose or didn't choose winding, stubborn roads.

No wonder you keep slipping all the time. No wonder the road lengthened and wound and even disappeared on you. And how will I help you get out of these so complicated places? You got lost to yourself and to me. How, despite all that lay ahead in the region we embarked on, did I lose you; how did you lose yourself?

"Ayelet— Aye, how can you even understand?" you asked. "You're all about control. You're always on guard, aware, thin; what do you even know about this struggle? You've never been in it, never experienced it. How can you understand the inner forces that pull you down so intensely you can't control it?

"Do you know what it's like to get up in the morning and hardly roll out of bed because your body can't carry you with all that weight? Do you understand how it feels to see food and not be able to restrain yourself, knowing it's stronger than you and will surely overpower you, no matter what strategies you come up with?

"I'm exhausted, disappointed, sad.

"I want to succeed, feel good, but instead, I run in circles. I watch it a little, but then not at all. And I struggle with myself and with food, and for now, it's winning BIG TIME!"

I was silent.

Perhaps I was mad at myself for not succeeding in guiding you without you getting lost. Perhaps I was mad for putting you on the defense due to my anger. But how can be mad at powerlessness, at weakness? Or am I angry at the hurdle itself and how it chose to take over you, of all people, and make your life miserable?

And perhaps, I was mad at you, for giving in to the obstacles along the way and slipping. Or maybe I find it hard when things don't work the way I want them to, and then I try to bend them according to my plans and thoughts. I know it's impossible. Everyone needs to follow their own path, and if they choose to get lost, I must enable that.

You know, Tamar, we never spoke about it, and maybe despite what we thought, you don't even have a choice. And that is what's making this struggle so sad. Perhaps there are forces in you that are more powerful than your own and they choose for you; impeding you. Those inner urges and desires, which are innate to you, may be stronger than you and your ability to choose.

I don't know. But I feel that it is hard for me not to be able to control—guide you as I would want or as I believe is best.

And moreover, I find hard that you can't control and guide yourself as you so want to.

The therapist's chair isn't necessarily a frustrating spot, but it seems that in the realm of treating obesity, there is something in the chronicity and difficulty of measuring achievements and successes that is burdening me.

The realization that success is something in the person's subjective realm is hard for me. I sometimes need the validation of concrete, clear indices to visibly and even scientifically evaluate the process. But, in the world of obesity, this is nearly impossible. Because therapeutic success isn't only measured by how much weight the person has lost.

There is stagnancy, sadness, pain. The immense hardship of bringing about change, and more so, maintaining it, makes the treatment frustrating and exhausting.

I feel that for me, aside from the patient's experience of disappointment and pain, there is difficulty in the

Ayelet Kalter

unattainability, the disappointment of failure. I think I belong to those types of people who love to conquer, achieve, win. And, in marking time like this, there is a sense of missing the target for me.

Perhaps it doesn't have to be a chair of frustration, but a chair of accepting the other and that which is unattainable.

What next? I believe there is a next.

First off, you're here. You haven't given up. You're writing again, connecting to yourself, and that's important. It's even somewhat of a beginning.

At least until next time.

It's strange, I wanted you to be able to make an accomplishment. I would be thrilled to know that you're feeling better about yourself. But, in your case, Tamar, and perhaps contrary to other cases, I find it hard to suffice with a good feeling or self-acceptance. It's important that true weight loss is achieved; a significant weight loss that will ease your health, and as usual, it's hard for me to make do with bits. What are five kilograms? A drop in the ocean.

And the therapeutic world is a microcosm of others' lives. There too, I want it all.

A lot and quickly.

Intensely.

Here too, I find myself at a loss.

Can it be that I'm giving up out of fear or dissatisfaction? Maybe because the process is unfolding differently than I expected, I chose to give up.

What is happening to me as a therapist opposite you, Tamar, if I become paralyzed? Am I finding it hard to listen to your needs? To see things differently, to move differently, to a rhythm that is different from mine?

I know that even though what is happening doesn't live up to my expectations, I'm not bailing out.

I'm in it.

I'm in it, though in my own way.

March 28, 2001

In the last two weeks, there has been a shift. Your commitment, presence, and wishes can be felt again. I'm slowly getting to know you. If you're happy or sad, satisfied or in a place of destructive self-criticism. I'm starting to notice when you're authentic or busy presenting a distant pleasantness while keeping rigid boundaries. I feel your eyes wandering around, inspecting the room and me, examining every feature in my face and body. It's hard to hide from you. You see the mask and what is underneath.

I feel rather all right with it. I don't need to explain, reveal. You're doing the uncovering. And it feels nice. And once again, the roles get muddled. But I pull myself together and assume responsibility.

You sat.
Watched me.
Waited.
So did I.
You said, "Aye, are there no more rabbits in your hat? Are there no more magic tricks that can do for me what I can't do for myself?

"Do you know how many times I've fantasized about going to sleep and waking up different; thinner, happier, lighter. Have you ever waited for someone or something to save you from yourself? I'm sitting here before you, after a long and draining work day. I make an effort to come, to talk about...and that's it? What about the effort to do? Why can't I find it within me? Where is it?"

What I wanted to do most is to get up and hug you. What else could I have given you at that moment? More advice, more insight? But I remained seated, debating where to begin, and remained silent. And, into that silence, the words broke out.

"Aye, I know it's not only will power. I feel like there are forces stronger than myself inside me, and it's like they're sabotaging me as if inciting me to fight against my war on food. As if deep down inside my body, there's some tiny creature that wants more and more and is lurking, waiting to seduce me, to make me fail. And he calls for me when I'm sad, when things are tough, and even when I'm just having fun. So, I never know when to expect him or how long he's going to hide before he rears his head again. So, I'm constantly on guard. Waiting.

"Actually, I think I'm wrong. It's not true, I don't think about him. It's as if I'm surprised by his presence each time. It's as if he reveals himself anew every time, and I am startled. I know he's always inside me. Sometimes more active and sometimes calmer, but he's always there.

"It's something a lot stronger than my will power, my decisions, my words. I even like him a little sometimes. He excites me, moves me, ignites my desires. Unexpected.

"Aye, it's not easy for me to be in this place, which is sometimes helpless, degrading and weakening. I, who is so controlling, strong, dominant. I fade before him."

I was quiet.
So were you.
The minutes passed, and we were sitting.
Silent.
The chatter that came from outside deepened the silence. Wintery sunrays signaled a sunset, the white neon light washing the disappearing red.

What could I have offered you? I know, as you do, that I have no bunnies in my hat. I have no thrilling surprises or exciting projects. I have a routine, a boring, banal framework, but a framework nonetheless. And I spoke of journaling once again, and once again I felt a little pathetic. I do believe that your ability to recap when you eat each day can be beneficial to you, but I know how hard it is to do that, and even more so, how hard it is to live in a constant battle against the urges and desires embedded in you, which powerfully control you.

Once again, I tried to enlist you, seduce you into journaling again—to connect to yourself.

You speak of pain, difficulty. And it's not only a physical experience that can be spotted and touched. Because this pain, Tamar, takes on amorphous, abstract and changing shapes in you.

I see it as the pain of stagnancy, lack of self-fulfillment and satisfaction in your life. A pain of crumbling fantasies, which you were certain you would fulfill in the course of your life.

Disillusionment.

And you?

Marking time in your routine; home, kids, work. You get your thrill from touching, helping and treating disadvantaged kids. Kids who, without people like you, would hang in opium dens, on streets full of crime. And you, with endless patience and a sense of vocation, protect them, show them warmth and love and try to impart some knowledge, a useful occupation, and a home.

But it doesn't fill you up completely. It doesn't utilize your potential to the fullest. Because you wanted to conquer the world, make countless discoveries. And instead, you're immersed in your own fatty swamp, which only perpetuates the pain and maybe even reinforces it.

Everyone has their own right path. And only you can find yours. I thought that by journaling, you might find it because journaling can take on different forms—each one and his journaling style, each one and his discoveries.

Just like Osnat's journaling was as vibrant and surprising as she is.

The morning began with taking Schnitzel, the dog, for a walk, during which I bought chocolate milk and a bun. It's my favorite chocolate milk that comes in a bag. I came home and sat down to read the newspaper while eating the bun and drinking the chocolate milk (like we used to do in summer camp.) The bun gets soft, and when you take a bite it simply melts in your mouth, and the chocolate milk drips out of it and wets your mouth with the cold, sweet liquid.

When I returned from you, Ayelet, at about a quarter after twelve, I started looking for something to snack on before I sat down to write my paper, because I didn't want to be very hungry while I wrote. I found leftovers of the chicken soup I'd prepared last week, and that was perfect, because even the noodles were ready in a container in the fridge, since I didn't have much time. I had to write the paper, right?

I heated up the leftover soup, which only had the clear broth, but the flavor of the chicken and the root vegetables was still very strong. After my belly got warm, it seemed like there was no way out of it, so I sat down to write. While writing, I needed some grapes in order to think and a little piece of Schnitzel that was in the fridge and needed refrying to make it crunchy, fresh and yummy again.

I finished the paper at about four (It's unbelievable how I procrastinate until the last moment, and then it takes me no time.) I went to submit the paper, and when I came back, Omer (a friend from school), who came over to write the English paper with me (which was also put off until the last minute), stood in the kitchen cooking lunch. He chopped a big onion and a few garlic cloves, two large tomatoes, potatoes, and chicken. Then he sautéed each one of the ingredients alone in olive oil. Finally, he mixed them together and seasoned it with Teriyaki sauce and garlic-honey sauce. To finish off, he broke two eggs that bubbled over the dish and gave it an extra-tempting look. We sat down to eat, and as strange as it may sound, this experimental dish was even tasty. For dessert, Omer grabbed a Popsicle from the freezer and made do with a cigarette.

At nine-thirty, I went out with my sister to the neighborhood café. I drank cappuccino and ate a slice of pie with crème patisserie (yes, yes), and unlike what I tried to do, this was the real thing: a vanilla crème with just the right thickness inside the pie, with bright red strawberries on top, devilishly sweet, simply divine.

That's it. The evening ended just as it began, walking Schnitzel, the dog.

Tamar is not the only one who hides her sensuality and sexuality under layers of fat.

Shlomit also created a huge, pouring belly for herself. It's like she is arguing with herself, but quickly falls plundered, defeated.

Shlomit came to me, like others, just to lose weight.

Fifty years old, divorced, bright blue eyes, and a belly.

The beginning of the process went smoothly. Shlomit kept an eating journal and lost weight. She lost about seven Kgs. and stopped. Seven Kgs. and nothing more.

A month, two, three, no fluctuation. With the overweight that she carried, we both knew it wasn't a physical hurdle or a plateau brought on by the body's refusal to cooperate. Another eight Kgs. and she would have emerged a new person.

Perhaps that is what scared her so much—becoming a new person. Is that what threatened her in parting with those eight Kgs.?

Together we tried to understand, to discover. And in this huge belly, hid the sorrow of loneliness, the romantic partnership she was missing.

It hid the pain of financial hardship, of conflicts with her adolescent children, who sucked every piece of private serenity out of her.

There were aches on an interpersonal level, from romantic relationships that fell apart and hurt her, the frustrating relationships with the kids, from whom she felt constant demands along with ingratitude for her efforts. And there was sheer exhaustion from the distressing, weighing down, burden of life.

And the walls came up over the years. Each wall was its own statement, as if she had built a safe haven for herself that no one could enter, a place of her own where no one could decide things for her. Only her and her body. Her with her large belly.

That is where she hides.

To my surprise, we just touched, and all the walls came crumbling down. We spoke to the belly and about the belly for hours. We tried to understand what significance it had in Shlomit's life.

Is it protection? Fear of sexuality? Is it fear of failure with the opposite sex and preparation of a perfect alibi?

Belly.

There's something cute and caressing about it. It has lots of space to store emotions. There's something soft and pleasant about it and even calming. Something maternal and feminine.

But with fifteen kilograms of belly there are also inhibitions, fears and anxieties. Such a belly contains pain and suffering of so called concession. Yielding.

Is this what Shlomit truly wants?

Is this what Shlomit truly summons into her life?

Is this the real Shlomit?

We tried to understand if she indeed wants and can part from this belly, which has been her companion for many years. I suggested she tried to talk to the belly and perhaps even write it a farewell letter. To try and say goodbye. I thought such as ceremony would bring closure aside from its symbolism.

And Shlomit wrote. And it wasn't easy.

My dear belly,

It's no coincidence we've spent so many years together. Sometimes you're a little flatter, but most of my adult life, you've stood out prominently. You can't be ignored.

The thought of having to give you up seems strange and even painful.

I'm used to waking up with you in the morning, wrecking my brain in front of the closet and mirror trying to figure out how to hide you and minimize your existence. I've learned to wear stretch pants with along shirt over it, or just a vest to hide you. I've learned to tie my shoelaces with my leg slightly raised, because it's hard to just bend forward. I've even learned to walk past the mirror and ignore you sometimes.

Besides, you know I'm pretty attached to you.

You allow me to eat as much as I want. There's lot of room in you for all the cakes I love, the cappuccino with the croissant and the yummy sandwiches. Thanks to you, when people ask me how I am I can always answer, "heavy," and "if I'd only lose a little, I'd feel better."

Thanks to you, I go to courses and men don't make a pass at me, I'm sure it's because of you, and that if you weren't around, I'd surely have suitors. This way I'm never anxious, because I always know that you're with me and taking care of me, and that no man would look at me anyway. Cause who needs a woman with such a belly? So then I'm not tense, not anxious and not even anticipating. These relationships are always disappointing and hurtful anyway, so who needs them.

And you know, this may sound strange to you, but there's something warm, prospective, calming about you. I feel at ease with you; you're reassuring, secure. With all the heaviness, ugliness and danger of illness you possess.

Besides, have you ever thought of how they would look at me if you weren't around?

No one will understand what happened to me and may ask, "Shlomit, how come you look so good?"

"We finally see your beauty, your radiant eyes." And I think I'll know what to say to that? I'm not used to getting compliments, and I surely don't know how to be in the center of attention. So maybe it's better this way, to leave you here with me for good. To stop trying to remove you, to accept your existence as a constant in my life?

And anyway, you probably won't want to walk away just like that. I think you've gotten used to being with me too. Going to sleep with me at night, getting up and smiling at me in the morning. You're used to dictating how I sleep, because with you I can't sleep on only my back or on my side. I'm starting to think that you quite like me and I guess I like you. So how can we say goodbye?

How can I go on without you; without someone like you backing me, supporting and protecting? Without having an alibi for my choices, my failures, my disappointments. Can you imagine me with a jeans and tucked-in shirt?

Can you see me dancing in events with a tight dress?

And maybe I'll have suitors, one of which may become a loving partner?

And maybe my daughters will also like the change and start to look at me differently? More appreciatively, more lovingly. Maybe that's what is wright for me? And I don't need to consult you or hear your opinion. You won't want to leave anyway, you won't want to give up your existence in my life. Maybe I owe it to myself, to try and see what it's like without you.

True, I find it hard to allow myself this "luxury," to spend so much money on myself. And maybe it's only an excuse and I'm just afraid?

But it seems there is no way around it, my dear. I want to do it. I want to try to look different, and maybe live differently too. I feel I'm ready for a change more than ever. And if not now?

When?

Later I; will be an old woman, and such a difficult operation will be dangerous for me. The recovery will also be harder, and I won't have enough years left to enjoy the change.

I'm sorry, dear belly, I feel that our partnership must end.

Despite the anger or sadness that you may feel, I ask that you wish me luck. Because I'm scared to death by the operation. What if it doesn't facilitate the change? And what if I don't feel better after it? And besides, what if the operation doesn't go well?

I owe it to myself.

So once more, my dear belly, I feel that there is also something positive about our separation. I feel that I am heading towards a new beginning. I'm excited.

Goodbye. I loved being with you; there were years where your presence in my life was vital and important. Now I feel the need to form other friendships, other feelings.

So…

Goodbye.

And the tears rolled.

From her eyes.

From my eyes.

Shlomit decided she could part with her belly, and it was a complex process. "Dieting" wasn't enough. It required invasive intervention in the form of surgery. Beyond the financial investment, it entailed many physical difficulties, perhaps even risk. But Shlomit was determined.

I was worried. I accompanied her with mixed emotions. I felt great responsibility. Yes, it was her decision, but I was there, lighting the way, implying, touching. Yes, she made it to the well; she decided to drink; but I showed her where the well was. I was afraid that aside from the physical challenge, there was a sea of expectations that might harbor countless disappointments. I worried about her ability to enjoy the change and allow herself to earn it. And at the same time, I wanted to believe that she would indeed grow and blossom from it. In a way that only someone who was immersed to his neck in this blubber swamp can be.

She underwent the operation.

Four hours. Her belly was slit, and a few kilograms of fat were removed. Stitches. A hard and complicated operation. Excruciating pain, immobility, catheter, special bandages, heavy elastic bands and six weeks of recovery.

This was plastic surgery, not bariatric surgery; it was meant to change the shape of the body and the distribution of fat in it. It was designed to significantly reduce the protruding, blocking belly—the belly that hid everything but itself.

I worried.

I felt responsible; I felt I was the guide. But ultimately, she did it. Alone. By herself.

So why did I feel so responsible?

I was even more afraid after than I was before the operation.

I feared the stage of awakening, of reality, or the scariest stage of all—confronting the..."no belly."

A week later.

Luckily, the recovery process is long and slow, giving one time to adjust to a new reality, sensations and emotions. Will a change indeed take place?

For years, her belly was on full display. What would her life be like without it?

I'm excited.

I sincerely hope that my strong desire for her to undergo a substantial change will not spoil it or rush it for her. Not everyone is as fast; not everyone reaches the "after" without first experiencing the "before."

I will make an effort not to want on her behalf, not to do for her, but simply support and wait, and have faith in her own ability to navigate herself in her new world.

What does this world look like?

What does a world whose view was obstructed by mountains and valleys look like once they are removed?

How does a person feel when he can suddenly see his intimate organs without needing a mirror? It's no coincidence that the belly protrudes between the breasts and the vagina. As if making a statement. Protesting.

It's like a smooth mountain you can only glide on, up and down, unable to reach the top.

How do you live without the mountain?
Without a place to hide behind?

And the process is slow as ever.

Coping with the pain, the awakening, adjusting to the change.

Shlomit took her first steps on the new journey she planned for herself. Everywhere she went, people noticed, saw and said, "You look wonderful, radiant."

Her body began to take on a different look, fresher and even somewhat inviting. The kids liked it.

And mostly Shlomit;

She was happy.

I remember the first pair of jeans with the shirt tucked inside. And the smile. Something profound happened to her; something made her livelier, less cumbersome. But that something had to be preserved. She had to learn how to live with. Love it. Accept it. And that is not easy. Because an operation isn't enough. It is an intervention that is outside Shlomit's control. Whereas now, she had to take back that control, be mindful, account for, listen to her needs, desires, and body. This amazing change needed reinforcement every hour of every day. Will the change awaken her to a different, more satisfying and happier life? Will it enable her to enter a new relationship, bring optimism and new beginnings to her, until then, smothered life?

Will Shlomit succeed? Years will tell.

I hope so.

I shall wait.

Impatiently, I shall wait.

March 29, 2001

It's been exactly two months; I didn't open these pages even once. The notebook was thrown into a corner; I didn't invite myself into it.

Even today, knowing that I will meet Ayelet tomorrow to read to each other, I procrastinated until nighttime. Only now, when it's already Friday, and I cannot escape any longer, I'm here.

I kept the notebook unopened and shut myself.

I shut myself against the tremendous pain I have felt in the last six months. Almost a physical pain. Lingering. Hardly letting go. Like waves in which I am drowning, coming up for air only to go under again.

The depths of pain alarmed me. I, an expert in suffering, scarred by death that came knocking at my door, and then retreated; I, who have obsessed and recapped so much; I, a veteran of the paths of pain and sorrow; I, who swims in shallow currents of invisible fear; I, who thought everything was under control and I was in charge of how and when.

I was stunned.

There is much darkness awaiting you around the corner, Tamar, and it doesn't taste well, so tonight I sweetened it with food and flight.

In the past few months, I've been more or less flying, leaving my consciousness. Oh, how good it is to return to the sweet, primitive, automatic split, one in which there is complete separation between the blind, uninhibited, mindless and emotionless eating and the feeling, mindful and humane one. Because in order to introduce mediation to the automatic, soothing, filling and intoxicating eating, I must constantly be focused on my awareness; in integration, a tremendous effort is made by my blemished soul.

As Ayelet put it, I took a leave.

I stopped relating to those extremely damaged places. I kept some form of eating that allowed me not to gain all at once the measly five kilograms I had lost and gained and lost and gained. As if I was in my last five kilograms rather than my first. I stopped making an effort to eat less and didn't give up almost anything in my gluttonous lifestyle, sinking into that addictive doing.

Lots of doing at work, all around. Overwhelmed by a tight schedule. I even gave up Meir in the last month. I didn't go to workshops and sessions. Because that's being. That is being with myself. And I only wanted to do.

Though being is usually restorative, healing, does me good, I didn't even want to be there. Because to be happy also requires a connection, and I didn't connect. I had a wonderful two months with a more stable mood, full of vigor and activity, a desire to see people and patience to others.

A true saint. How lovely.

And the pulse of dissatisfaction was dimmed, its volume faded. And I didn't make an effort.

But it was temporary. It can no longer suffice.

Because otherwise, what's so horrible about living with this weight? Pay its price, and earn some peace. But I need more out of my life. I can no longer live on false and borrowed peace. I can no longer make do with tiny islands of mediocre happiness.

I'm searching for more. I want to be happy.

I'm lazy with Meir, too. Because there, when I make an effort, I manage to access my center, and there are partial peace and happiness there. In the last month or so, I've drifted away from Meir as well, because allowing myself peace and happiness is an effort for me.

And the road is long.

As far as weight loss, I don't have the option to stay the way I am. Staying that way means sinking, retreating, giving up the hope for happiness. Well, happiness is a big word; I'm not betting it on this in any way, but I think that if I manage to do something about it, it will bring me closer to serenity. It seems to be a highly dangerous zone, because as soon as I step in it, I sink, and I don't really get to confront it. Only a little.

I can't settle for not touching on it at all or constantly touching on it. I need to find a way to touch and live, a combined, complex way. yet to be paved. It can simply be a path. I have to return to this path.

Not escape.

Not escape anymore.

Because there is happiness in the end or at least fragments of it. And peace. It's no fantasy; because I've experienced peace with Meir a few times.. and I know it's all there. On this path— in the center.

Just be there.
Be there without fear.

Ayelet, A-ye-let. A-ye.
The invisible, transparent curtains between us have been removed.

There was some closeness, and within this tango, we both stepped back.

I'm startled by the intensity of pain caused by touching myself, startled by the intensity of exposure before Ayelet. And Ayelet, who also touched herself slightly, in our last session when we read and didn't talk, maybe she got startled. In addition, maybe not, but she lifted a screen-curtain.

She can only do it intimately, and she can't be intimate at all.

She's attractive and interesting to me.

But I don't know the everyday Ayelet, and she doesn't know me.

It's as if we started from end to beginning. In short, it intrigues and attracts me, yet also deters. She's becoming important to me. There aren't that many like her. It's threatening and alluring at the same time. Part of my motivation for continuing with this adventure is some deep, unfound knowledge that, with her, it can move somewhere. That with her, it can work out. Maybe it's the functionality, vitality, frankness and ambitiousness (wow) that she radiates, which help me fill up with strength.

No Ayelet.

I'm not banking everything on you. But it's interesting. Had I lost interest, you could not have continued. And maybe this lack of progress isn't vital for now.

And we arrived back inside the tunnels
Flooded with salty waters
And the bitter foam came into the mouths of the submerged.
And those who managed to float it
A slice of air touched
Their bluish body.

For a fraction
Crystal butterflies sowed in me
Curls of ribbons,
The flutter of wings,
Morsels of sweetness.
And then,
Drowned.

In a reddening bog
The defeat of lions
Depressing desire
Trembling
Heat
Of their insult.

And for a fraction
I believed.
(Ayelet)

During my work, I have come across many exceptional romances with food, but I believe Naama's romance is one of the most fascinating ones.

Naama, sixty-five. Strangely divorced.

She lives with her daughter but is visited by her ex-husband on a daily basis.

He visits her home every day at the same hour. He stays for an hour, talking incessantly about his work, himself, and she serves as a kind of sympathetic ear. She doesn't share her world with him. Every so often, they go out on different events together, but every night, he returns to his other home, his other woman and her two children.

Every day, Naama waits for him at the designated hour.

Naama has been coming to my clinic consistently for two years. Her pleasant face cautiously discloses some bitterness, like a snail peeking out of his shell, testing to see if he's allowed, if it's safe, and fearing he might get hurt if he takes his head out.

Naama is confined to a demanding, stressful set of commitments, which involves endless giving without boundaries and a complete obliteration of her true needs. She finds herself controlled by the needs of others (her father, children, ex-husband), and is inattentive to her own needs. The main need she dares feel is the need for food, mainly sweet things.

On the one hand, she discovers maturity and readiness in herself, and on the other hand, she is aware of her childish side. For example, she plans her binges, many times, just waiting for her daughter, the gatekeeper, to be out of the house. She plans how she is going to sit and eat the sesame candy, the chocolate. How she will feast on sweets.

Sixty-five years old. Fragments of her femininity are still somewhat shy.

Only she.

She will decide what to eat, how much, how, when. Only she.

Since she never gets to choose in any other area; she is controlled by others' demands. But here, she is running the show. Here, she decides and sets the rules. And it's even fun, pleasurable, exhilarating. There is something soothing about this secrecy that strongly impacts her. She decides she controls.

As if there is some victory to this eating that says, "You think you know and decide, but here, with food, only I know. Only I decide and set the rules."

But the "power struggle" only begins here; it grows and intensifies in the non-verbal dialogue with her ex-husband. There, even with food, she is no longer in control.

Her husband always brings her special sweet treats he receives at his workplace. Lots of them. His usual ritual is to ask her, "Did you eat? Was it tasty?" and she, conditioned since long ago, nods. Eats. Everything.

She has never thrown away anything, never given these "sweet golden treasures" to anyone else. Because she's afraid of what might happen if she does.

Perhaps he would stop bringing them to her and give them to his "other wife"?

Perhaps he would be mad?

What happens if he is mad?

His anger frightens her, paralyzes her. His anger makes her recoil.

What if she refuses?

If she refuses, maybe he will stop coming.

And then what?

She will be alone, completely alone.

What about herself?

What about her own wishes?

So, like an "obedient girl," she eats. She leaves nothing, she throws nothing away, and she surely doesn't share.

She fills her body with two kilograms of sesame candy, fine chocolates, dates, in quantities, and everything is delicious, going deep down inside her.

What would happen is she willed for herself what she truly needs and feels?

Warmth.

Love.

But Naama gives in.

He brings, she eats.

He asks, she gives.

She doesn't dare break a ritual that is so false for her, or perhaps it isn't false. Perhaps by sustaining this ritual, she actually gains a lot, even if it is tidbits he throws at her. She holds onto every tidbit and takes it deep into her body.

She settles for what there is. No caress, no touch, no fulfillment, and certainly no feeling.

And eats.

Everything.

The only place Naama dares to express her feelings of anger and pain is in the food, and it continues to fool her. Comforting and compassionate at first, it turns quickly into devouring, deadening, painful.

Her "husband," who has been living with another woman for years, and all the while visiting her for symbolical purposes; her "husband," who never legally separated from her, is signaling his serious intent to return "home." And it's not the first time. They have been through this before.

He leaves, continues to pay rent, and when he gets tired of roaming outside, he returns, without asking her. After all, it's his home, he can do with it and with his spouse as he pleases, but there is no true feeling of love there.

And what about Naama?

It's irrelevant. No one is interested in her wishes and feelings. She learned to hide them, bury them deep.

She learned to eat instead of being angry.

To eat instead of feeling.

To eat instead of talking and standing up for what she wants.

She is afraid, dependent on him, his money, his existence, his anger.

Above all, and despite being aware of all his emotional shortcomings, she needs him and can't give him up. Perhaps through him, she still feels valuable? After all, of all his wives, he always returns home to her. He loses interest in them and comes back home. She is the only one he never loses interest in. She is sad, trapped, angry at him, at his emotional handicap, at the fact that he sees her as an object. You use it when you need it. When you don't need it, you put it away.

I suspect that she is mainly angry at herself, at her powerlessness, her inability to express her anger. To rebel.

Naama is frustrated by her inability to listen to her true needs, most of which are true friendship, a sympathetic ear, understanding, trust, and credibility. The desire to be with a friend you can lean against when you're tired, cry next to when you're sad, that would be there for her, contain her.

When all that doesn't exist, she eats, a lot. She doesn't dare to express her feelings, to open such deep sounds that would bleed and hurt.

The thought that he may invade her life and move back in with her horrifies her. Having to share a bed with him, report her every move, play the temporary role of a wife, all these drive her crazy. She can't be with him, and she can't be without him.

And where is Naama today?

Naama lost about 14 Kgs., which is 18 percent of her body weight.

She isn't thin, but she feels better. Since the emotional issues in her life continue to dictate her eating behaviors, she

The Weight of Happiness

continues to waver. Indeed, less chaotically, but she fluctuated by 6–8 Kgs. To her credit and thanks to the process, she has never returned to her original weight. And we are talking about an almost five-year process.

What characterized the therapeutic process she underwent is her ability to carry out a dialogue with herself and with the food she chooses to eat. She has learned to ask herself why she is eating before she does, whether it is physical hunger or emotional hunger, if it is instead of feeling anger or frustration, or more so, a difficulty in expressing those feelings.

Naama also tried to find out if when hungry, she chooses to eat because that is what she really wants, depending on her needs and likes. Throughout the therapeutic process, she tried to discover her true needs and even respond to them. Together, we tried to make her confident in herself to believe that she knows how to identify what she really wants for herself. This process started with food and continued to other areas in her life. It mainly touched on her interpersonal relationships.

I think the change was predominant in her relationship with her husband, who has yet to decide where he belongs and continues to maneuver both worlds. He continues to visit her home on a daily basis.

Within the enduring chaos of her life, she finds herself less controlled by his needs, more daring and attentive to fulfilling her needs. She no longer eats for him. She no longer eats to please him. Her fear of him has diminished and made room for inner power that enables her to place clear boundaries between him and herself. Between his needs and her needs. And she eats differently. She manages to maintain her weight so she feels better about her body.

Yes, there are good times and hard times. But overall, she is in a healthier, more contented place. She understands and even accepts certain situations in her life that would once drive her crazy. Today, she has learned to live with them somewhat peacefully.

Her binges have waned in frequency and intensity. She has even managed to throw away 1 Kg. of sesame candy and not panic over it. She dares to express and feel her anger and aggression. I believe this, too, has been a relief for her.

Naama tries to be mindful of herself and her needs, navigate what she gives from a more peaceful place, less compulsive and less guilty. And, when it gets to be too much, she allows herself to rest a little. She may not be "thin," but she is in a different place with herself.

And she feels good there.

At least for now.

April 4, 2001

The notion hit me like a thin, cold ice pick penetrating my ribs. Like a strong, burning ray of sun blinding the pupil that was used to darkness for so long.

She might not even realize this, or she may, but have not yet said it to herself. I saw it in the dull look of her blue steel eyes. I saw it in her distraction, in the tiny nuances at the corners of her mouth.

She lost interest.

Her patience ran out.

She, who conquers new summits quickly and scrupulously, at an unbelievable pace. She, who has no tolerance for the average, the slow.

She, whose name is synonymous with pragmatism, operability, productivity, and success. Has lost interest.

It is bothersome, taxing, boring, nothing is shifting, the words have gone bankrupt, the magic of the onset is gone, there is no bottom line, are no results. The success measures have backed away in shame.

The Project has failed; moving on to the next one.

The Project Queen, at least four or five simultaneously.

There is no satiety in this emaciated, ascetic body. Instead of food, she fills herself up with projects. And, as with food, it never satisfies her, no matter how successful she is. This I know and can understand. Success only satisfies me temporarily, too. And, if achieved, no problem, but not at this crazy pace of course.

I felt like a string was torn. She just wanted me to leave. She was impatient. There was anger in her icy eyes. She invested precious time in her tightly filled up schedule written in large, childish letters.

And I, whose time is precious and running out, too, am treading in place. Wallowing in the murky mud, which isn't for her. When there are puddles to cross, she gallops over them, or rushes easily, marking her light step in them. Onward.

She asks me if I have given up. If it's the end for me, but what she's really telling me is that it's the beginning of the end for her. It's her projection. I'm not even there, and I have told her that in the past.

She dried up all of her creative ideas. Contained, supported, was present.

The "we" and "we lost weight" and "we gained." She pulled out all of the bunnies from her dietetic hat, but nothing budged.

And it's no longer "we." She's estranged and cold as ice, and it's me, who doesn't have any bunnies in my hat. And when she asks me what would I do differently and what I feel when I don't succeed, I have no honest answers for her or for myself, and I won't go into any manipulations, though I'm pretty good at that as well.

But not there, not with Ayelet.

Now, I'm alone with only the very end of that glove Ayelet threw at me seven months ago. This white glove is slipping, and it's my responsibility to catch it and ask Ayelet to not let go. No more words; it's time for your actions, Tamar. This is the twilight in which you're weak at; you must start to walk. No more Ayelet, no more the tough and almighty one. No one owes you anything, no one will do it for you, and no one will take your wallowing for very long. Your charm diminishes and fades, and you, you'll take action, or you'll remain behind again.

No more chances left.

She turned west
Where dark ships sink
Heaved their guts
Into
Uneven waters.

April 5, 2001

You chose to bring me what you wrote yesterday.

I think I almost shed a tear.

I felt the pain of fighting an endless battle, crawling along without reaching anywhere significant. I found it hard to be in the passive position forced on me. I was especially frustrated by the lack of tangible results in the form of kilograms.

You're right when you say that I have a hard time with the lack of success and progress. That slow, not-goal-oriented pace is hard for me that it's tough for me not to be able to control and manage things. How can you control and manage another person, especially when he chooses to get lost?

You're wrong about my perseverance. It's hard for me, that's true, but to give up?

Not here.

As long as a patient doesn't give up on himself, I'll never give up being there for him.

Besides, I'm a firm believer that only a person who stops walking, fails. As long as a person moves on, despite a succession of failures, he will reach a better place for himself.

So long as he tries, I will try with him. I will be at his side, for him, and I suppose a little bit for my sake, too.

I have no doubt in your sharp outlook and insight, Tamar. And I know that by virtue of you being a therapist, you examine me up and down, leaving no surface uninspected. But how much of you do you project on me?

Is your feeling that I've grown tired of you or given up not a reflection of your feelings about yourself? Your anger, desperation and disappointment with yourself?

And I'm the mirror.

The container.

I'm not disappointed.

I'm sad.

Not because the journey failed, I'm sad for you, Tamar. I feel your pain, and it's piercing like an ice pick. Sharp, penetrating and burning in strange places. And you're wrong, Tamar, I do know. I do talk to myself and wonder.

I don't give up.

So long as you wish to talk, I'll walk with you.

Always at your side, for you,

Not instead of you.

April 15, 2001

Our last meeting, where we read to each other everything we had written in the weeks that had passed, was lopsided to begin with. Blue sky, smooth, glistening sea, the vibrant, alluring hubbub of Friday, and the two of us.

You and I.

And what's easier than sinking in a sea of mundane, flowing chitchat? I directed it that way. I steered the session to the beach. An escape? Believing it's possible or simply wanting to cruise it? It was an unnecessary loss, not appropriate at all, not for you, Tamar, and not for the process. And I don't think for me either.

Café, the aroma of food, the clanking of coffee mugs and the clamor of people. You and I at a table, alone, but not at all, really. Surrounded from every direction. Chatting, noises; how can one even talk, work?

Perhaps that's exactly what I wanted when I brought us to the beach, the sand, the sea, not to know, not to confront and deal with the difficulties. Not to understand the nature of your stagnancy that sabotages your health and your feelings toward yourself.

And what does such a session look like?

We talked about movies, books, a little about the kids, a little about nothing, and a lot of silence and sound of the sea.

We enjoyed it, but I felt guilty.

We both felt how we were running away from touching, confronting, digging at your stagnancy, Tamar.

At my feelings toward it.

At your inability to arrive for sessions.

At how you run away from yourself.

At the high sugar, which demands an immediate weight loss or medicated treatment.

At my frustration for the lack of progress.

At my difficulty continuing to contain and encourage you in the low and high places where you wallow.

So, we went to the beach.

And there we had water and sky to talk about.

And there was the ice pick that sliced your soul and made you acknowledge that you're alone in this battle over yourself, and no matter how much water and sky surrounds you, you're alone.

April 16, 2001

Ayelet suggested we meet outdoors.

The thought that crossed my mind was, "Why does she want to leave the therapeutic setting that we all learned is so important?" But I told myself, "She's the therapist; it's not your place."

We arranged to meet on Friday at a beach café.

A table under the hot sun, close to the entrance. Endless traffic of passersby. Merriment, kids running around, guys and dolls, noise, heat.

Too-intense colors of ocean blue and blinding yellow.

Exposed.

Everything besides intimacy.

I realized even before we came that it was a mistake to come here, but I let Ayelet lead.

Why did I agree to come?

Why didn't I tell her what was going through my head when she offered to come here?

I like coming here with friends, with Nadav, to breathe the light-blue scent that rises from the sea, to give in to sappy sunsets and to eat. What business do I have coming here with Ayelet?

With Ayelet, I'm in dark, black, still, blurry places.

It was almost surreal.

We ordered breakfast.
And I'm in distress.
I want to wolf down everything: aromatic, puffy buns sprinkled on top with black cumin and coarse salt, a steamy omelet, an assortment of fatty cheeses, lightly salted salmon, thinly chopped salad, yellowish butter, fresh guacamole and homemade jam.
What a torture.
How come I have to eat in front of her?
We chitchat, exchanging opinions and impressions.
And eat.
Ayelet focuses mostly on vegetables.
She is full-on self-control. She taught herself to love what is healthy and non-fattening.
She eats very little bread, no butter of course, and refrains from eating a lot of the fatty cheese, smoked salmon and jams.
I'm being a good girl.
Diet coke instead of freshly squeezed orange juice, and I leave food on the plates and bowls in front of us. Even some of the buns remained in the basket. I eat about half of what I would have eaten had I come here with friends. As it is, I ate about four times what Ayelet ate.
Ayelet said, "I'm waiting for the muffins that come with the coffee."
I also know the breakfast here, but I've never thought of waiting for the muffins; you eat what you get, and if the muffins arrive, you eat them, too.

Not with Ayelet; everything is calculated.

She already knows how many calories she's eaten, and how many are in the muffin she awaits.

Everything is under control and thinking one step ahead.

How can you enjoy food when you count every bite?

Poor thing.

But, when the muffins and coffee arrive, I don't touch them. I'm embarrassed.

How does she kill this lust by counting calories off by heart? (She must have something like a cash register in her head that counts and calculates every bite.)

It also sounds like an eating disorder; a healthy eating disorder.

Shrunken.

In control.

There's no joy in Ayelet's eating; it's no great fun eating with her.

We drink coffee; my eyes follow sadly as the half-full plates are being cleared off our table.

I'm not used to eating this way.

I'm not one of those fatties who doesn't eat in company, then binges later in secret.

I eat openly in dinners with friends, with family or alone with Nadav.

And a lot.

Friends like going out to eat with me or to eat at our house. I'm a good cook and am knowledgeable about food. Food is a festive, joint celebration.

My more miserable eating is the non-festive one, which doesn't bring me pleasure, like at night time in front of the TV, when that void creeps in and occupies space. I don't enjoy that meaningless food eaten offhandedly.

It holds no joy.

We finished the coffee, and Ayelet suggests we take out the pages and start working, reading to each other what we had written in the past months.

It didn't seem right to me, but I couldn't say anything to Ayelet. I let her lead; it's so unlike me.

Since when do I let anyone lead me? With all the noise and hubbub, the blinding sun and the deep blue, we read to each other what we wrote.

I wrote a little. So did Ayelet.

It's no coincidence we wrote a little. I wrote a little because I wasn't really present.

I wasn't present in any process in the last few months. I took a step back, I didn't really bring myself to it or do anything about it. Nothing significant happened in the sessions with Ayelet or in my life.

For at least two months.

I think Ayelet is also feeling like nothing much is moving with me.

It was pretty horrible to read the intimate lines we each put on paper within this ruckus.

I felt so exposed, so unprotected.

If I had distanced myself from the process, I now wanted nothing but to escape.

Ayelet Kalter

I wanted to run away from there, from this surreal scene.
I was mad at myself for agreeing to be led here.
I was mad at Ayelet.
I wanted to vanish.
A miserable meeting.

May 1, 2001

I'm worried; the sugar levels are skyrocketing to over 200. You're weak. You know what the accumulated damage is, damage to blood vessels, the complications involved.

I'm powerless. Frustrated.

How long will you sabotage yourself, your body, your soul?

What else needs to happen to make you stop self-destructing?

You're big, fat, suffering.

Afraid.

Tormented.

Death awaits you in every corner, real and tangible.

And I, I want to help but I can't.

I want to make you healthier but I can't. Parting with the fat is hard for you; you're hanging onto it.

Could it be that you have given up on your life? That you have chosen not to fight? Opting to let life run you rather than you run life? Will your power remain buried under your fat? Your power is centered on your ability to help other but yourself.

I stand on the side.

Watching.

You take care of your parents like only a few know and can, with gentleness, care, and love. Despite the fear and hardship, you're there, in your entirety, like only you know how.

And at work?

You're like a tireless turbo engine. You take care of the kids because there's no one to care for them. You fight for them and win for them, so as not to allow them to sink into their miserable reality of drunkenness, violence, theft and drugs. You're one-hundred percent there, giving. It's your vocation.

And at home? To Nadav, to the kids, all of yourself, which is a lot.

So, there it's possible? Only when it's for other people?

Could it be that all this giving empties you, and then food comes in as a filler?

I don't know, Tamar.

I only know that I worry, that I'm mad at the weakness.

I think that giving up is what's hard for me, especially when a person chooses to give up on himself.

Perhaps we can look differently at the thoughts that are harmful to your manner of eating? Some thoughts almost immediately trigger a binge without being preceded by preventative or delayed thinking.

And it is the thoughts we can control at times. Because if we learn to identify certain thoughts as problematic, and know that every time they penetrate our head, they may harm us, perhaps we can push them away. As soon as we become familiar with them, we can perhaps hold negotiations with them and maybe even prevent them from offsetting an eating binge.

I shall illustrate it by using a number of examples for irrational thoughts:

- "Either I do this diet perfectly, or eat as much as I please."
- "I either show up every week having had no binges, or this whole treatment is just a failure."
- "If I ate high-calorie junk food that isn't acceptable on a diet, like pizza, the whole day is ruined."
- "I gained two kilograms on the second week of the process. I'll probably continue gaining every week."
- "When I was young, people picked on me because of my weight. If I gain weight, it will probably happen again."
- "Although I didn't binge during that last event, I felt like I did, and therefore it makes the day a failure."
- "If I gain one kilogram, everyone will notice."
- "Everyone will notice I gained weight. I won't be able to handle it; therefore, I shouldn't meet anyone."
- "I had a bad food weekend, so I may as well stop watching. I can't do it anyway."
- "No one spoke to me during the party, probably because I gained weight and I'm fat."

Does it ring a bell, Tamar?

Gather your strength, Tamar. Use it to take care of yourself, your body, your soul. It's hard for me to witness your endless pain. You're running away from it, numbing it with food and resentment about the fat. And then, you're busy with the binge and not with what triggered it. And it may be easier, so you think because it's a concrete occupation, but in reality it's no less difficult. Because you're sick, cumbersome, having difficulty wearing clothes, going on trips or dancing like you love. You suffer from the heat.

And I see and remain frustrated.

And you know, and remain fat.

May 3, 2001

The unfortunate meeting at the café distanced me.

It distanced me from Ayelet.

It distanced me from the track I was starting to follow in tiny, first steps.

Ayelet abandoned me.

She abandoned me to the sun, the sea and the sand. I felt so unprotected.

How could she initiate an outdoor session in such an exposed environment?

How could she let us sit opposite each other and eat, then have me read such intimate lines about myself with strangers around us.

She made all the mistakes a therapist can do.

And I'm that much angrier because just when I finally allowed her to touch me, treat me – just when I've given in to it – I'm back at my usual position – the objective professional.

After all, I know a thing or two about therapy. And as a therapist, I know we both made all the possible mistakes.

How could I let Ayelet lead me there?

I, the opinionated, the bold, the leader.
I agreed to be led. I greed to be treated, to give in.
And where did she lead me?

Go find me, Ayelet.

May 5, 2001

You're angry; I feel it, and I know it.

I think there is truth in your words, but I feel like you're holding onto that event as an alibi, Tamar.

Distancing yourself from yourself started before our session at the café. Your various excuses for fading in and out of the process existed even before that. So let's be honest with ourselves and not blame everything on that unfortunate session at the café. I sense your feeling of betrayal very strongly. That strange feeling as if I'm abandoning you to the sun, the waves, the strangers. Not protecting you, the framework, the process.

And I?

I knew it even before I parked the car and before we sat down.

But I was paralyzed. I continued to lead us to the corner table under the blinding sun, the aromas of breakfast in the air and the busy waiters rushing by us.

We sat down despite that, and we tried to carry on a worn-out small talk despite that. As if I didn't feel or know that the whole session was fundamentally wrong.

And as you pulled back, so did I.

From confrontation.

From the painful truth.

From that stagnancy.

Yes, I'm the one that must assume the responsibility, and I assume it, all of it, but, Tamar, let's not continue to wallow in this place and hang your entire lack of progress and escaping on it.

Come, Tamar.

May 7, 2001

I'm overtaken by a sense of duty once more that I have when that happens to me.

I'm fully enlisted, wanting for you. It's taken a lot of energy from me.

Yesterday, when you came, I felt it throughout my body.

Huge, yet somewhat defeated, scared.

I examined your heavy body, your rolls of fat, refusing to release these choking rings. I saw the sadness reflected in your eyes and felt how all my words and wishes for you passed by you, gently caressing your hair, body, and a little bit of your soul, without penetrating you or reaching you.

Yes, you've been named a diabetic.

You take medication, but you know as well as I do that it's not a lost cause; that if you truly rise to the challenge of your body, you can heal it.

You can.

But will you dare touch it? Embrace it?

Or will you continue fighting it, wounding it until it collapses and drops at your feet like a casualty?

I felt the panic grabbing your throat; you wanted to speak, but you choked.

Slowly, the broken, fragmented words came out.

"Aye," you whispered, "I'm t i r e d. I don't have what it takes to fight. I don't really believe in myself anymore. I see the plagues coming, and I can't really confront them. I can wrangle myself for a week or two and then crash. I don't follow through. Not with sports, not with eating less, not with reducing the sugar in my daily food plan. I know what it takes so well, yet I can't do it.

"Aye, I'm terrified.

If the sugar continues to skyrocket, what will be then? I'm afraid of gangrene in my leg, vision, and circulation problems. But I can't. What about my kids? How can I look in their eyes and admit that I knew but couldn't watch it? Besides, do you even know the consequences this has? In daily functioning, in my inner feeling?

"And I see it, helpless. Could you believe that, Aye, me, me, I'm helpless!

Defeated—by myself."

I hurt for you.

Yet I said, "Tamar, I feel your distress and fear very strongly, but I know that if I sink into these feelings with you, I won't do you any good. You say you're tired, depleted of energy and sincere strength to motivate you. But we can't stay in this position even a minute longer. I thought that perhaps instead of being angry with yourself or looking at your body like a punching bag, which does you no good anyway, you could try to begin to love yourself, your body. View it not as an enemy, but a partner in life you can talk to, touch. Even befriend a little.

There are no winners in war, Tamar."

It's scary.

I feel your dead-end. I know that if you shift even a tiny bit, everything will look different. You could forge ahead. Peel away the fat wrapping your body like a bear hug.

May 8, 2001

My sugar is very high, but I'm not able to lose weight anymore.

I can't even continue writing the food journal, though I know it helps me maintain control on a daily basis. I went to the doctor because I realized I couldn't go on like this. She sent me to do more serious tests, and I started taking Glucomin.

That's it.

I've been named a diabetic.

I keep escaping this title, denying my ailments.

When the year started, I went for a comprehensive checkup so I could receive permanent status at my new job.

Transferring from one employer to another requires a comprehensive physical.

The last time I took such tests was nearly twenty years ago.

The tests came back, and I was called for a meeting. They didn't want to grant me permanent status due to my screwed up tests: diabetes, high blood pressure, "cancer patient in remission." I'm not in remission from cancer; it's not a break. I know I'm healthy, that the cancer won't come back.

What about the diabetes and high blood pressure? I never took them seriously. After you get cancer, none of the routine ailments seem serious.

Now I'm getting on medication.

So, it means I'm really sick.

One pill a day.

I know that if I lose ten kilograms, the diabetes will disappear.

How do I do that?

May 13, 2001

I thought you would show up on Friday morning filled with motivation to carry on.

The fact that you hadn't called yet is a warning sign.

I hope you haven't sunk into the abyss again.

Yes, you went on a field trip with the students for three days, filled with anxiety and stress, but you returned, and everything had gone according to plan.

And I waited.

Waited for you to come.

And you, Tamar, chose not to show up.

What does not showing up on Friday mean for you? And not only did you not show up, you asked Nadav to make the phone call for you. A laconic message, "Tamar won't be able to come today; something urgent came up at work."

Urgent?

What could be more urgent than you, your health, and your needs? Why are they taking the back seat again? Or is it simply easier, more comfortable this way? Anything but touching yourself. Giving into giving, work, forgetfulness.

I refrained from calling; I didn't want to force myself on you or coerce you into the process. I felt that I needed to allow you to continue escaping until you decided otherwise. You need to do it your way, at your own time. Although I'm impatient. "So muster some patience, Ayelet," I told myself. "You have to for yours and Tamar's sake."

I wondered how much time you would take off. Could it be that things became a mess a while ago, and you're tired of coping, ashamed, and fearing my reaction, my expectations? I hope not.

It's important for me that you don't run away even if it was a bad week and you did not meet your or my expectations.

Not from me and from yourself. I'm aware that sometimes I project a certain level of expectations that may pressure the patient, and I try to avoid that, but right now, all I know is that all I have left to do is to wait for you.

I'll do that.

May 15, 2001

At least you're consistent in one thing: in running away.

You don't show up for sessions, with all kinds of excuses of "I'm very busy at work," running to take care of your parents, and all those mundane things that can be used as an alibi. Neither you nor I buy these excuses. You've obviously entered a cycle of binging and self-deception.

"One more day, and I'll straighten up."

"This week I'll be good, and then I'll go to the session."

But all this self-convincing only deepens the gap between you and yourself. Pushing you away from being able to reorganize your eating.

Because from a perception of "all or nothing," you won't rise and harness yourself for real unless you hit rock bottom.

I don't expect you to be flawless or keep to a perfect diet of 1,000 calories a day.

All I expect is that despite the hardship, you continue to come. That you continue confronting yourself even if it's painful and frustrating.

Tamar, who said that you have to crash in order to evolve? That you must first devour thousands of calories in order to regroup? And who said that only the "impeccable" have a reason to show up to sessions?

All I'm trying to tell you is that if you succeed in showing up to sessions, despite it all, it might not be so messy. Or if it is a mess, perhaps it will be more moderate. There is still a difference between 2,000 calories and 5,000 calories.

You know, Tamar, the willingness to look at the difficulties often minimizes them, whereas running away from them only amplifies them into a large snowball that accelerates and chases you.

I feel like I am tired of chasing you. Explaining, being empathetic and attentive. Do you think I feel comfortable? So what if I know that this is the right thing to do therapeutically? Does it make it easier? I also have my limits. Just know it's hard for me. I'm disappointed; I'm certain that you're missing the momentum of the illness big time. It's hurting you, destroying you. You got saved by the skin of your teeth.

And this sugar that signals every other day also has something to tell you, but it's as if it doesn't concern you, doesn't scare you.

Therefore, if you choose to wallow in yourself, I'll let you be.

I'll give you all the time you feel you need.

I have nothing left but to watch and wait.

This is the only way right now.

When you called yesterday and I told you there was no appointment for you, because you didn't schedule one, and I didn't do it for you, you didn't ask why; you didn't fight. I think you were even relieved.

I know and feel when a patient wants me to fight for and with him. You didn't indicate that, Tamar, not even a hint. I suppose you felt comfortable with the void that settled in. You essentially told me, "I'm not here." All I have left to do, aside from feeling it's a shame, is to wait for you to reappear.

I'm waiting.

May 17, 2001

I can't bring myself to Ayelet.

I can hardly open this notebook and write what is happening to me.

Something went wrong in that whacky session at the café.

I can't bring myself to myself seriously.

I started with the pills, and I thought it would shock me profoundly.

I thought it would lead me to do something.

But the opposite happened.

The sugar evened out.

The pressure was off, so I don't have to lose weight.

I'm healthy again.

What's healthy?

Health comes from creation. Meir says that if you're connected to creation with love, you're healthy.

Lately, I don't feel truly connected. I don't feel connected to creation, I don't feel any light moving between me and creation, and I don't feel like my body and soul are connected.

I'm ignoring the body.

I'm switching to end-of-the-year mode and bailing out on myself as far as eating.

I'm bailing out on myself and on Ayelet.

Perhaps this is the place to introduce some waves of optimism?

My clinic does not only witness stagnancy and sadness. It has a lot of light, too. Real successes, not just in the positive feelings inside, not just acceptance and compromise, but absolute victories—huge ones.

I met Rona in December 1988.

Twenty-two years old, pretty, with magnificent curls and many excessive kilograms. Every morning, she would drink a glass of orange juice for health; eat a bowl of cereal with milk, for pleasure; and a salted pretzel, to be full. This was just the beginning of the day, and she already had 800 calories under her belt.

At lunchtime, she realized she had hardly eaten that day and would splurge on a roast beef sandwich dripping with mayonnaise. And, if that weren't enough to satisfy her, she would cook pasta with mushroom and cream sauce at home and finish off with a large Cheetos snack bag in front of the TV. The early afternoon hours included a chocolate bar filled with chocolate and another one filled with coconut. Years later, when the candy bar turned into an ice cream bar, I would see it daily on her eating journal pages in pairs.

I was at the beginning of my therapeutic work, full of optimism and belief that I could lead the patient to actual slimness. I wasn't aware of the complexity of the process, the extent of frustration, especially throughout it.

A young woman weighing close to 80 Kgs. is a lot, no matter how you look at it. And there was a real challenge here. Back then, I was still giving out diets and food plans that included exact instructions on what to eat, when and how much. We would plan it in detail, trying to understand what would be best for her, what she wanted and mainly what she could. Rona followed the instructions.

She would arrive weekly at 7:20 in the morning by bus and on to work from my clinic. Disciplined, consistent, and mainly filled with the desire to lose weight and look better.

And she indeed lost nearly 14 Kgs. over eight months and looked amazing.

But the euphoria didn't last long. Pretty soon, she began to put on weight again. A year later, she weighed 77.5 Kgs. No plan and no diet helped. She simply couldn't gather herself together and cope with giving up food and the deprivation entailed. Food, which had a major role in her life, took center stage again. She ate indiscriminately, uncontrollably. Mostly junk like snack bags, pretzels, cereal, and other high-calorie snacks.

Depression, disappointment, desperation.

We didn't give up. I think we dared to look at things differently. Be happy that she didn't climb back to 80 Kgs., understand that she's highly influenced by her interpersonal relationships and that her entire emotional constitution easily tips accordingly. We acknowledged that every emotionally charged situation ends with uninhibited, maniacal eating.

I think we both realized that after years of overweight, it's hard to all of a sudden become a "hottie." A hottie has a different social status, different needs. And maybe Rona wasn't ready to be there yet?

We pondered this, but we continued on our journey, slightly staggering, slow, one step forward, one step back, but never giving up. One week, she lost a half a kilo, and the following week she gained it.

It was tough.

She ate and tried to keep to the plans we set for her, trying to make them fit her, her desires and urges. Soon enough, I stopped writing food plans for her because I felt they were useless. Eating and needs change on a daily basis anyway. We sufficed with her writing down what she ate, and there were weeks where even that was hard for her to do. But one thing was clear to us both: she would show up consistently and not run away.

One time, Rona's mother called me angrily and said, "You're wasting my daughter's time and money! She's not losing weight anyway!"

And I, a beginner dietician, was partly terrified, partly hurt, but answered politely that I asked her to wait patiently and let her daughter manage her eating and cope with it by herself.

And so it was. Rona showed up consistently. On the bus, in the rain, in the heat, despite her weight fluctuating between 73–74 Kgs., she managed to see the achievements and didn't give up. Rona noticed that she had slightly more control over her food, that the binges lessened, both in frequency and in intensity, and that she didn't go back to her scary weight of 80 Kgs.

Some may ask, what is the difference? The 74 Kgs. is also overweight. True. But, in the realm we deal with, you learn to accept the non-perfect. You learn to enjoy the small achievements, too.

In 1992, Rona managed to go down to 64.3 Kgs. for the first time. She looked wonderful. She enjoyed and loved herself like she hadn't for years, but she could not keep this weight down for more than two months. Once more, following an emotional turmoil over a failed relationship, she climbed back toward the 70s, where she wallowed for about six months.

Had we drawn up Rona's weight graph over the years, then within those ups and downs, she was still at a much better place. If before, when distressed, she would gain weight to around 80, now a low point for her is around 70.

The struggle continued, and Rona didn't give up. Another six months went by, and one day, she dropped down to 60.6 Kgs. This happened in October 1992, almost four years after we first met. The weight continued to trick her and she settled with desperation, between 68 and 70. She rested there for close to two years.

The changes occurred in 1995. She met Amichai and felt good. For the first time, she felt serenity in her relationship. And so, as the relationship deepened, she slowly glided for about a year and a half, until she reached 59 Kgs.

By September 1996, Rona reached 58.5 Kgs.

She was happy as can be.

Gradually, her weight stabilized and settled between 57–58 Kgs.

The more the relationship developed, the more her weight stabilized, as if it were her body's natural place.

Today, seven years later, Rona is married happily with two children.

She still looks amazing and weighs 57 Kgs.

I see her from time to time, once every two to three months, just for follow up and reinforcement.

For years, she showed up every week consistently, until we were certain she had reached a safe ground. Only then, did we begin to schedule sessions further apart, excited each time anew at her success and ability to manage her eating in a way that enabled her to maintain a stable weight and feel good with her body and eating behaviors.

What in all those years finally enabled Rona to reach a better place? First of all, perseverance. She showed up regularly and didn't drop out of the process, even when everything seemed hopeless. She didn't run away from herself and remained present even through the painful, frustrating stages.

The persistence alone helped whatever damages she made be under some control; not everything was lost. Indeed, once we started working together, she never reverted to her original weight.

What characterized Rona in her long journey she took was that she worked at it.

She wrote in her eating journals, confronted, coped. During the journey, she learned to manage her eating differently; to think, plan, have priorities, understand what controls her, what makes her tick, what is right for her to eat, choose and even enjoy and feel satisfied.

Beyond the therapeutic process and the change she adopted in her way of thinking and behavior around food, I think her ability to develop a supportive partnership that was right for her, deepened and reinforced her ability to maintain her achievement. Those places she would fall into due to emotional pain, disappointment, and frustration, which she couldn't handle, many times, and ended in binges, were redirected at some point to the relationship that filled in the voids and created a strong, genuine source of support for her.

There were many struggles and slips along the way. There were weeks where we pre-planned what she would eat down to the smallest details, and other weeks when we went along with her inability to act. We tried to listen to her needs, abilities, likes. In recent years, Rona has acquired a whole new eating language. She thinks and acts differently. She has assimilated an earnest change in herself both cognitively and behaviorally.

Therefore, her weight changed too.

For good, I believe.

May 20, 2001

Tomorrow, you are scheduled to arrive after an absence of more than two weeks.

I'm busy talking myself into not showing my disappointment and anger that may erupt unwillingly. I'm busy diffusing my level of expectations.

I know it will be hard for you to show up tomorrow.

To see me. you, the weight.

To experience failure all over again.

And I'll be tired, I know that.

Of you, of the virtually foretold chronicle of watching a little and then unleashing a lot. From the world of fat that is so resistant to therapy, the damages it brings and especially from doing nothing about it. To watch, see, and not be able to drive you forward, in an attempt to watch, reduce quantities of food and peel off some of the mass of fat cushioning you.

And I'll be sad.

I know it.

But I will be here.

May 22, 2001

Another rejection.

You called to say you weren't coming.

My first feeling was disappointment; I know what those cancellations mean.

In other words, "I'm not here, I'm not interested."

After the disappointment came the anger.

I make such an effort for you, and you cancel just like that.

How can you do it to yourself, destroy your health with this eating and fat? Don't you care about your body, your family, your life?

After the anger came the sadness.

For my powerlessness in helping you, for your inability to help yourself.

For knowing that suffering. For the loser feeling that takes over me in these situations.

After the sadness, came the surrender.

It's strictly yours. I do everything in my power for you, but I can't be responsible for your choices.

When you want, come, I'm here.

And, after the surrender, it finally came down to me. Here I dared to feel myself. The self hidden under the therapist's hat. After all, it's impossible for these two hats—me as a person and me as a therapist—not to mix, even if a little.

Feelings of hurt rise slightly, unsure if they are allowed to reveal themselves outright.

When I sense that the person before me is under duress, suffering, and pain, and that I may help him, even if a little, I immediately enlist myself, without verifying if it's right for me. And then, I expect more, am more exposed and vulnerable.

I want this for you, Tamar, both as a person and as the therapist.

So then, your escapes are confusing, disappointing, hurtful.

There is frustration.

I'm aware of your landmines. Your difficulty handling my expectations of you, and your expectations of yourself. It's hard for you to disappoint me, but it's especially hard for you to disappoint yourself. I may be wrong, and you're fine with yourself. You eat, dose off, hide the raw feelings. But with me? You know you can't hide from me. I see, ask, and challenge.

You escape to your demanding job, which sometimes threatens to swallow you whole. And I guess for you, it's good.

I'm carrying a dialogue in which I'm the only participant.
Where does that lead us?
You?
Am I here alone?

May 31, 2001

You didn't entirely escape, only a little.

You didn't show up for more than three weeks. An annual field trip, hospital visit with your parents, heavy load, and fatigue. But it seems to me that you mainly "didn't feel like it," "was over it." Journaling, coming, making an effort, giving up all kinds of beloved foods, facing emotional distress. So, you simply didn't come.

I was hoping the illness and the fear of sugar levels (for which you started taking medication) would enlist you and affect your eating behaviors. I was hoping that fear would shake you up even a little.

But no.

You managed to watch, calculate, listen to your needs, and plan your food for two to three days, but only for those days. Then you soared to your consuming routine and "forgot."

"Forgot" to write.

"Forgot" to plan.

"Forgot" to come.

Now, as you sit before me, a little embarrassed, willing and unwilling to acknowledge the damage you accrued during the long vacation you took, I wondered what to say.

I asked how you felt, your thoughts, expectations. You told me about the difficulties, the nights filled with corn puffs, the greasy food at work. You spoke about your work colleagues and the challenges in your interpersonal relationships, and about the weak, lightheaded feelings when your sugar was raging. You expressed self-disappointment at skipping sessions and food journaling. But you felt you couldn't do any differently. You didn't want to face up to what you ate, how much and why. You simply wanted to enmesh with it all, perhaps even morph into the chaos you had brought on yourself.

You were leery of reprimanding, anger, criticism and a massive hike in weight. You felt cumbersome, lethargic and sad. You sat before me with that heaviness, fatigue, and desperation. We both knew that as long as you evade, you would keep running in circles, because it's always hard.

There will always be more important things to tend to.

You apologized, explained, but we both knew that these were all excuses.

I tried to be with you, understand your hardship. I didn't criticize or judge your choices.

I only listened.

And after you blew off steam and got mad at yourself, and mostly once you felt relieved by coming back, I tried to find out how you felt about getting weighed.

Yes, there was chaos and disorganization, and there was surely no reason for you to have lost weight, but I thought that weighing you would mark the end of one chapter and the beginning of a new one that might be different. I wanted to show you that you have done a great deal by finally bringing yourself back here and that I believed in your abilities.

The weight surprised us both—110.5 Kgs.

Though it seemed to you like you were going through another eating binge, and with all the chaos in your food, you didn't gain weight, and that was enough to draw strength from. Because it may be that your feelings of guilt for not journaling, not showing up, not being connected, colored your eating in far darker shades than what it really was.

It's true that not all the damages have manifested, but there is still the imminent threat of weight gain. The good news is that if you enlist yourself now, there is a chance that this increase won't happen because your awareness and watchfulness will prevent deterioration. So instead of wallowing in what was, we can perhaps move forward to a new beginning.

June 2, 2001

I managed to bring myself to Ayelet after a long time. There wasn't much joy in our meeting. I didn't miss her; I didn't miss the setting. I went because I felt that this whole thing was starting to slip between my fingers. I didn't really want to let it go. I didn't really lose my desire to do something about this, and I knew that if I succeed, it will only be with Ayelet. I'm not really in it; I feel it; I don't have the same intimacy I had with Ayelet, either, but I don't really want to check out.

I went to the meeting and got weighed, and I didn't gain.

I didn't write down my food and didn't watch very carefully, but I guess I didn't binge that badly. Maybe because I've been so busy lately.

So at least I didn't gain weight.

That's something.

June 12, 2001

The journey is progressing slowly, if one can talk about progress.

It travels in many directions, if one can talk about going somewhere.

It goes around and around, if one can talk about turning.

Everything seems to get lost.

To who?

To me?

She who is searching for purpose, aim, profit and loss, is asked to move back and forth, with no plan, no future. Many times, without even a present.

Stagnancy.

Where?

With the one who finds it hard to be.

With the one who always needs everything to be clear, planned, in control.

How am I with vagueness?

What happens to me when everything seems stuck?

June 16, 2001

To connect to that journal of mine, to the food, to Ayelet, is a nuisance.

It's a nuisance because I'm in a crazed, action-packed mode at work.

It's the end-of-the-year frenzy, but the atmosphere is fun and our activities are successful.

Maybe I'll feel somewhat satisfied just by that. Maybe I'll get to enjoy it for more than a minute.

Ayelet.

Wait for me. Don't run away. Make do with what I can give now.

I'll be back sometime.

Can you be patient?

June 21, 2001

Tamar.

How long will you fade in and out of commitment as you please?

You don't seem to be able to remain consistent. To persevere.

You're not really gaining anything from the process.

It's all in fragments. A little of everything. Never the whole thing.

Somewhat connected and somewhat not.

June 25, 2001

Meir helped me connect to my serenity joyfully. Open. Light.

The shadow of the curtain plays with the sun across the bright floor when I lay down on his mattresses. I'm fully relaxed after a treatment in which I visited other dimensions. After Meir's treatment, I stayed for the workshop. I had time to hang out and experience the wonderful energies flowing through my body after he pressed all the pent up points and made the depth of my soul vibrate with healing.

I was bathed.

Clean.

And we spoke about opinions in the workshop.

If you're truly present in your life, if you live in full presence, without checking out, with full being, you can give up opinions. Because today, I can have one opinion, and tomorrow it can change.

What does it mean to be present from the inside? To separate between my inner presence and everything else, work, family. Experience myself as separate from my environment and be present in myself. Maybe being present in myself means also to connect to my body.

My poetry notebook is gone. I left it. I didn't take good care of it.

And I'm hurting. And I'm mourning.

We spent a miserable weekend at a hotel in Tel Aviv. A cheap weekend. And, as always, I took my poetry notebook wherever I went. In the evening, when we sat at a café on Hayarkon Street, the entire street emptied all of a sudden, and we heard many sirens of ambulances and police cars.

As time passed, it became clear it wasn't just an accident. Rumor spread that there was a terror attack at the Dolphinarium. We walked back to the hotel, staring at the horror on the TV screen. We didn't feel like doing anything. I sat down on the balcony and wrote.

The following day, on Saturday, we went down to the beach. It was desolate. The shock of the attack left us without much desire to do anything special. We returned home rather early. Two days later, when I wanted to write, I couldn't find the notebook.

This time, unlike him, Nadav did a final check in the hotel room to see that we didn't forget anything, but the notebook hid under the weekend newspapers. Nadav tried to inquire at the hotel, but they said they didn't find anything. Three years' worth of poems were written in it.

David, who led the writing group, always told me to type it on the computer, to save it. "It's no good having everything written in a notebook," and of course, I never did it.

I was ashamed to mourn this loss.

How can this compare to the youth whose lives were lost in the attack?

I secretly thanked God that this was the only loss I had to bear.

But, as time passed, the pain set in. Especially at my poetry group, after David's horrified reaction; he thought some of my poems had to be published.

I didn't feel like writing and didn't even buy myself a new notebook.

Ayelet shared my sadness.

She bought me a new notebook and wrote that every end if a new beginning.

A cliché, but true. I was moved by this gesture.

Ayelet has a lot of kindness in her.

I told Meir about the pain of my loss.

Meir said that losing words is like losing opinions.

Meir said the poems passed through me. I had already done what I needed with them. So don't hold on to them; don't hold on to matter, don't hold on to words.

Be grateful that this poetry went through me.

I don't need it.

I don't need it written own.

I'm trying to breathe at the loss of words.

June 28, 2001

I floated in the past months on a joyful creation full of gentleness, I guess because it involved many tears shared by everyone. Tears of saying good-bye to our graduates and end-of-the-year blues.

In these two months, I functioned almost unhuman-like. Very little sleep, many hours of work that involved physical and emotional effort. I wasn't particularly connected to this business of food, of eating. I had no time for it, I wasn't focused on it.

Had I not been a compulsive overeater, I could have lost a lot of weight, because I exerted a lot of energy compared to myself. Some of the time, I ate only when I was hungry, but I still ate a lot, and bad food.

If I had vegetables or healthy things in reach, I could have filled myself with them, but I didn't take them with me.

So, it's true I didn't gain weight, but I could've used it to lose some.

I wasn't in touch with many parts of me during this period, and of course, the first part to go is my fat self.

During such a period, I don't even feel fat. I'm light, floating, disconnected from my body, I'm all-mighty, I achieve, I get to everything, I'm driven.

I have no body.

No worries.

But I don't tend to the body either.

It's not a deliberate sabotage, but it's carelessness.

Spontaneous, a childish life full of intensity and feelings that send you into tough places.

The connection to these kids, from a deep, invigorating place.

It's funny to call them kids. Sometimes, they're bigger than me.

Huge Fifteen- and eighteen-year-olds.

Their ups and downs in the years I've been with them, their stormy, difficult lives, the relationships that constantly change, constantly evolve, (how they test my trust) all that creates deep emotional tornados that fill me and empty me all at once.

And I'm neither with the body nor with the food.

I eat out of habit of quantities and things lying around, out of habit and lack of thought. I wasn't preoccupied with myself in the past two months, and that was wonderful. I experienced a lot, I immersed myself fully in endless giving. It feels so good not to be preoccupied with myself, my body, the food, the fat.

So good.

July 1, 2001

So where are you, Tamar?

Cruising?

I went away.

And you followed suit.

As with any vacation I take, you take one, too.

I traveled to the Dark Continent, to Madagascar.

A friend, a local tour guide and myself. Just the three of us across the land where most of its inhabitants are busy with the daily task of survival. In large parts of the continent, there is still no electricity or running water. Most of the nutrition is based on primitive agriculture and a barter economy. The term "diet" is used only for matters of health and the supply of vitamins and minerals. Most people don't have the privilege of relating to their body weight, the shortage or surplus of a few kilograms. They aren't free to ponder the essence, needs, desires, frustration or concessions. They are busy living. They are busy fulfilling their most basic, vital needs for survival.

You traveled to more familiar places, of binges, falling into oblivion in a sea of food.

And we didn't travel, nor are we traveling.

We are stuck.

For two weeks, I was free of the weight, commitment, and caring for my patients. I was busy with myself, my enjoyment, my serenity. I enjoyed being alone, I enjoyed the mostly uninterrupted nature, the Baobab trees with their exposed trunks and heavy gaze, the clear sunsets and mainly the seclusion.

Apparently, I was not the only one enjoying this remoteness; you also led yourself far away, but differently. You have been vacationing for a long time now, ever since that scary hypoglycemic attack.

And you were actually quite okay with us continuing this hiatus. A little longer to get lost in the sea of endless freedom food provides you. You wanted more of that no-holds-barred taste. Eating without boundaries, checking out, escape. From yourself.

Hiatus for you doesn't just mean thinking what to eat, how much and when. It has something far more seductive about it. It has freedom, which is wonderful in itself. And you feel good there, but you also feel bad.

And I wonder.

Do I let you splurge until…and let you pay the price?

Part of me wants to allow you the pleasure, to run wild and abandon your body. Why should I be the bad guy? Will it help at all? Another part of me wants to take the back seat, wait in the corner, and adopt an argumentative attitude. You want freedom? Fine. I'll give you as much freedom as you want, and let's see what that does to you and what you will say then.

And sometimes, I wear the authoritative therapist's robe, who assumes responsibility, navigates, and decides. No more. Even freedom has boundaries, and we must create them. And I stop, pick up the reins, hoping I will be able to stop your horses galloping down the slippery slope into the abyss. And I did exactly that.

The main problem lies in the fact that I am only seemingly in power and control. In reality, I'm limited and constricted by your desires and wishes. If you choose to continue this hiatus, any boundaries I might enforce shall fail. Any framework that I may create shall fall apart. The question is how to enlist you? How to get you involved, caring, acting and account for yourself? Cuffs won't do it. You could be on hiatus with handcuffs. Even when everything is seemingly locked, s cage and lock in the form of journaling, weighing, and soul searching isn't enough.

Only you are with yourself. No one but you can enter.

Tamar.

I feel like I'm falling asleep. I feel parched. Like a carriage with a driver, reins, wheels, but no one to pull.

No one.

August 20, 2001

It's been so long since I opened the journal.

I promised myself to do it on holiday, and watching the Mediterranean shine in blues and greens, I breathed peacefulness.

On my quietest week so far this year, I tried to connect.

Ayelet says I've been on hiatus from myself for a long time as far as my commitment to my eating.

And she's right.

After the end-of-the-school-year frenzy was over, I fell back into a slow, routine month of work, and finally, I had the opportunity.

At the end of June, all the pressure at work subsided, and Ayelet went traveling. Had she not traveled, I would have managed to gather myself and get back to working on myself with her. She left, and I took the opportunity to rest and not get into any commitment.

Thus, the holiday slipped between my fingers, and I know I have to come back with strength to lead a new year.

And what about strength for a new year with Ayelet?

How do I manage to lead such a complex organization as the one I work for, yet find it so hard to inch my very own carriage forward?

It's been almost a year. Move, move forward.

September 9, 2001

I didn't write a thing.

I didn't feel the need to.

Or maybe I simply had nothing to write about.

You were there, but not really.

You came every so often, but you were on some long hiatus because you really did nothing that indicated a dialogue with the food or awareness of it. You didn't write, you didn't think, you didn't plan, and you didn't ask yourself what you needed.

You touched on it yet you didn't.

You wanted yet you didn't.

And I? I thought it was best to reflect to you how I truly felt. To show you that even though you come, you really don't feel part of the process.

And I wanted you to know, Tamar, that I'm not involved in your choices.

They are yours only.

I'm tired.

I'm no party to this game. I don't assume responsibility, I don't fight. When you want, I will be there for you, but only when you want. When you stop telling yourself why not. When you truly enlist yourself for yourself.

Because a fat Tamar is known and familiar and even comfortable for everyone. Because Tamar, with her impressive personality and abilities, isn't threatening when her shortcoming is announced in the open. It's easier with flawed Tamar, for you and for those around you.

Everyone can see you're not perfect; you're overweight, cumbersome, inflicted with ailments. Tamar has defects, too. And that is easier to live with forgivingly. To accept, to not be envious, to not want to be like.

So why bother losing weight?

Sometimes, desperation is so convenient.

So, let's stick with it.

What is all the compassionate talk about the essence of the fat, its role as the protector in your life, the guard, an alibi, a wall, cause and effect? They will never lead us to change or surrender because we'll always be sympathetic as to why you're fat. Why you need to eat right now. Why you're not free to practice caution.

And then, we're left with dozens of excess kilograms.

And I?

How can I be mad?

At weakness, powerlessness, giving up.

A year later, and we're running in circles around ourselves, not really going anywhere. Yes, you're here, and that's an achievement. You're not running away. But we get that already, we've been here before. And it's really not enough when you weight over 100 Kgs. The fact that you lost nine kilos doesn't really allow you to rest on your laurels. You still need to drop at least another ten kilos before we can perhaps see the effect on your blood tests, blood pressure, and overall well-being.

And this little-big step is so hard for you to take.

It seems to me, Tamar, that you wear dozens of hats.

One wide-brimmed, one has feathers and chirping birds, one is pinkish with sun and waves. One is a serious top hat, one is a simple cap with no frills, you can whistle with two fingers between your lips and even get a biker's helmet with sparkly sequins you can hide in.

And you switch hats without prior notice, sometimes wearing one on top of the other or a few at once. It's one of the things that fascinates me about you.

But, with all the depth and spirituality, you move in circles. With all your knowledge of yourself, your fat pushes you away from yourself. Because there is a great distance inside you that you can seemingly touch, but not.

You touch a lot, but there are hidden places you don't dare reveal, and they are left dormant, uninhabited.

You don't approach them.

They are off limits.

The fat protects, removes, enables not to know.

A year has passed.

Should I give up?

Giving up entails significantly heavier implications, even more than those dozens of kilograms you are carrying. It means giving up on yourself. This in itself can throw you into worse places. The hike in weight is endless, and the self-destruction capability is surprisingly powerful, so why test its limits?

Tamar, do you understand how frustrated and helpless I am?
Do you realize how much I want this for you, for me?
You, the large and present. Mighty as always.
You touch me.

The gates of heaven open up before me.
Carefully selecting their words.
The finger of God points forward.
Accusing.
I look down.
Pondering.

The purpose of therapy.
Quantitative results.
Profit and loss.
Benefit.
Isn't the process itself enough?
No! Not here. It's not enough. Not for me and surely not for you, Tamar.

A year has passed. We both continue to march. We don't consider stopping, though we aren't sure where the road leads and what will happen on this curious journey.
I don't know how to stop marching, I can't.
I'm here, Tamar. I'll keep on marching. Even alone.

Perhaps you'll want to rest a little (as you have done more than once), but watch me continue to march, gather strength. Join.

And so I go onward.

September 14, 2001

A year ago today, I embarked on this adventure.

I thought I knew the script ahead of time, more or less.

After all, it is my eternal pattern of an excited beginning, and when routine sets in, I lose interest and leave. But here something else happened; he routine is indeed frustrating, but I don't leave.

First off, though there was optimism and interest at the start, I wrote religiously but didn't lose weight significantly.

Meaning, I didn't really succeed in giving up food, although I know that there was hardly any binging involved.

That is, I came, wrote, got in touch with myself on the issue of eating in an almost scary manner, but I didn't really manage to change the behavior and management of food in a way that would allow me to shed a large number of kilograms.

I've been trapped in my huge body for so many years, and it's been ten years since I managed to look and feel really different. When I got sick, I lost nearly ten kilograms due to the nausea and treatments so I could wear a lot of things. When I was sick, I felt more shrunken, more contracted. I think it was a subjective feeling. It's true that I lost 10 Kgs. and everyone around me responded, but externally, the change wasn't significant.

It was really the inner feeling.

I began my path with Meir. His treatments, spiritual workshops, working on myself, my inner peace, and really the peace of the entire family. Ironically, although I had cancer, although I let poison into my veins that destroyed my body, I felt clean, purified, light. I didn't even hate my bald head anymore. Even that was a sort of purification. With all that yellowish complexion and the circles around my eyes, I was radiant. The discovery and connection to Meir cleansed me. And I allowed the toxic solutions to intoxicate me for a while, to cleanse me from the inside. There was even serenity sometimes.

But at the same time, it was hard to enjoy the body. I was afraid of it, I felt it was leaving me. Unable to protect me, neither I did it. And, if I couldn't protect my body, why should it protect me? Only after I betrayed my body, did it betray me.

Even though it shrunk a little, and I started eating healthier and differently, these ten kilograms didn't stay off for too long.

And the feedback around my losing weight didn't do me good as usual.

First, I'd apologize immediately and say, "it only looks like it because of what I'm wearing," or "I lost about two kilos, but that doesn't count."

I notice that almost always when the scale shows a significant loss, I immediately stuff myself that day.

But what happened here, with Ayelet, is that when the honeymoon was over, in which I hadn't lost much, and the routine set in, where I had to harness long-term commitment, I didn't escape this time.

And that's what nearly always do. At some point, I cause the people who treat me to leave me, or I manage to walk away from them and part as friends.

This time, it didn't happen.

That is, I failed in most of my recent sessions with Ayelet. I'm hardly able to lose weight and don't manage to always write. There are periods when I disconnect with this failure; I take a hiatus, as Ayelet puts it.

At times, I do get in touch with failure. Every week, I show up, a sign of failure is waiting for me. And connecting to this place isn't easy for me because I can't handle failure; I've hardly ever failed in my adult life.

And when I was about to fail, I fought tooth and nail, making sure I got a second chance because failure is rejection. It means, "You're not worth it."

And with failure I cannot exist, because I'm always worthless in my own eyes, not as good, and always needing to prove myself. I cannot simply be.

For me to be significant, I must always be active.

There is not contentment in just being. There is no peace of mind.

And my size is such a testament to that.

I'm a failure.

A visible failure, unhidden.

A failure that everyone, including myself, is forced to see and be with all the time. It's true that in a safe, familiar environment, I'm not attached to it all the time, but the taste of failure is constantly on my tongue. A bitter taste that contracts the tongue pores to an unripe dryness. Dehydrated. Barren. No matter what food passes through it, it cannot cover up the taste.

To stand in front of the mirror of failure is like being transparent. It's nonexistence. I'm erased. I have no raison d'être in failure. My security is so extroverted. Like my fat. Inside, I'm so small.

Nonetheless, although these weekly sessions strip me naked in every sense, and it would have been typical of me to give up and run away, I still show up.

Against all odds, I don't know why and how, I continue to come. It's not easy finding myself repeating the same exact ritual week after week, facing Ayelet and trying to figure out with her what else can be done to enable myself to take this chance, this opportunity. Maybe it's because I know this is the only chance. Maybe it's because I know that here, inside this terrible, inexplicable, scary pain, where I run out of words and definitions, which I'm so good at, lies the real work I've never done. Not really.

Because being without connecting to the pain is no longer an option.

This pain indicates internal burns. It happens when I ace my journal, or in my stronger sessions with Ayelet when I allow myself to truly be. It immediately emerges. You don't have to summon it. It floods and paralyzes me, weighing me down. The intensity of pain surprises and scares me every time. Most of the time, I manage to numb it in different ways. One of them is through food. But, if I stop and just connect to myself regarding food, it attacks brutally.

Ayelet Kalter

Maybe this size is something much simpler. Maybe it's just a bundle of behaviors I've adopted, bad behavioral patterns around food, which might have come about from a purely physical place.

Maybe it has no spirituality involved.

Maybe it's all substance, and what we're looking for doesn't even exist? And maybe I just can't behave any differently?

And I'll stay this way, live my life like that?

With all the suffering involved.

How can I accept that it is a bundle of behaviors? How can I be larger than life, but so small when it comes to food?

I wish I'd be left alone, I wish I could leave myself. I'm so tired.

I so want to go to sleep and wake up to find it all gone. Simply shed, be without it.

Maybe I need to love and accept this body first, and then I can give it up.

Yes.

I'm grateful to my body for cooperating with me, for destroying the death that was lurking in it and choosing life. And we were both left to continue this embodiment. Maybe when I was sick, and death grew and multiplied inside me, my body and I actually allowed us to recover; maybe that was the only time I loved it or was grateful to it. I had a powerful serenity that left me when I recovered.

I don't know where, how and when I will be able to touch this scary pain in a useful way, shall we say, from a constructive, nondestructive, healing and recovering perspective.

Right now, all I can do is show up and not give up the idea.

And Ayelet.

Ayelet manages to be there. I sense her disappointment, the knowledge that a year has passed and so little has happened. And although I lost nine kilograms in total, I've been stuck for a long time.

With all that, Ayelet is still there.

And I guess this is why I'm able to live with the failure right now instead of escaping to other obvious successes at work, in daily life and in general.

October 10, 2001

Being there all the time. Sympathize. Please.
Is that enough to move you forward?
Isn't that what is keeping you stuck?

November 2, 2001

Be.

Be with things.

How I push myself into a corner. The tests that will undoubtedly turn out normal threw me back to my fear of dying, to realizing how fragile life is.

And I'm still at the side of the road. I still haven't chosen one. I'm entertaining the idea, I'm pretending, superficial on a spiritual path.

I'm talking about Tamar, I'm living her symptoms.

To be inside her is another story.

To be inside her is to put myself first. To be connected in each moment and remember the work I have to do for myself. To understand that things originate from the inside. To understand, I have to take care of myself.

To understand that everything begins and ends with me. There is no one else and nothing else. To be on a spiritual path is to know for real and to internalize that reality is what I make of it. Reality is in the choices I make from what life brings. And that everything life brings is for a reason.

But am I truly there?

Telling myself and acting on it too?

In order to do it for real, I must attend Meir's workshops every week, listen again and again, and practice. I need this constant coaching because the spiritual path doesn't come easily to me. But when I'm truly connected, breathing with things, not letting all the drama in, I feel much better. And, if I go to Meir regularly, I have much better energies, and my spirit has a peace of mind.

But of course, I don't do all of these. It's an effort. An effort that entails traveling, money, and as always, I don't put myself first.

And as I neglect the spirit, so I neglect my body. I don't make an effort to take care of it, exercise, eat right. Lose weight...lose weight...lose weight...lose weight...lose weight...lose weight... lose weight...lose weight...Why am I tearing and feeling pain when I insist on writing this again and again?

But that's not all.

I haven't been able to internalize the separation thing Meir spoke of. I don't really know how to separate myself from the other. I never learned how to be side by side with another, how not to be all-encompassing.

Mainly not with those who I hold dear to me.

I'm going to Meir because I took some time out on Friday afternoon for myself. And I'm traveling to Rehovot.[29] I'm going for a treatment.

---

[29] A city south of Tel Aviv, Israel.

It's impossible to leave the city, and I've been idling for more than half an hour. There are cops standing and directing traffic on the highway. They blocked the road. An explosive? A turned over truck? God. Why can't I get to Meir?

At five to two, I turn onto the freeway when my appointment starts at two. I don't understand.

Why? I've already freed up my time for this.

So why can't I make it to Meir?

Everything is jammed. I feel the jam in my windpipe. Everything is blocked. Shut.

One big jam.

Instead of going to Meir, because my appointment had long come and gone, I travel west and reach the sea, the port and sit here.

And all this in order to get in touch with myself and write what's already been written. You've earned yourself along with the sea.

And when I call Meir to tell him I'm stuck in a traffic jam, he says, "Be happy. Be happy you're healthy, that there's nothing wrong, that your tests are fine. Be happy that you didn't make it because it was probably your lesson for today."

And what is the lesson, Tamar? What is the lesson by not arriving at your appointment and getting answers from Meir? And what's the lesson in coming to the sea to be with yourself?

I need to search for the answers within me.

Why is the road so hard?

How do I learn from all these lessons Meir has been talking about in his workshops?

I'm still a lousy student.

Ayelet Kalter

I paved you a path
Steaming
Smelly,
Seeds of shame.

A vane of life
Scattered
Mist,
In cracked termite hills.

The Golem
Danced
In the puddle
Cushioned with dream
Butterflies

And you were left
In the nothing.
Alone.

(Ayelet)

November 15, 2001

To be filled from the inside, not the outside

Fragments of eroded sun
Turning in my belly
A washer
That cannot
Get rid of the dirt

A thing crack
Becoming visible
Between the music box full of surprises
And my life.

I completely lost myself in countless hours of work. I allowed it to take over me. My sugar levels went up immediately, and I drowned.

I gained two kilos, and it seemed I had once again contracted a horrible cold and fever, which has only let go of me in the last two days after using medication.

I'm exhausted both emotionally and physically. Work is harder, more crammed, volatile, flooding, drastic, fast-paced.

Only if I tend to myself and regain my place, will everything around me become saner because what's inside if what's outside and what you give is what you get? And I'm giving more avoidance of myself, my body, my well-being needs. And I get more and more dramas, earthquakes.

Today I counted. I have a day off, and in four hours, I had twelve phone calls from work.
How can you take time out of yourself this way, Tamar?
And the same goes with my health. I still don't take the time out for it, not really.
Not with physical exercise and not with food.
I'm incubating.
I can't really gather up the strength to truly take care of myself.
It's so easy for me to take care of everyone else around me.
I don't really love myself, I almost don't.
In fact, most of the time, I quite despise myself, and this wheel turns endlessly, with no end and no beginning. Only when it opens and becomes an ascending spiral going upward, will the light penetrate it.

How long will Ayelet wait for me before she breaks?
I keep things on a low fire, not taking real action.
There are only our relationship and my pretty consistent arrival. Sometimes, I manage to write, and sometimes, not.
In any case, whether I write or not, it doesn't change my food quantities. I eat a lot. All the time. Not in binges, not sweet things, and not particularly fatty either. But a lot of food, most

of which is pretty healthy actually, cooked without oil, but still huge amounts of food.

And my sugar levels are high, not dramatic, but high.
And, naturally, my agreement with the doctor didn't hold water.
I asked for a three-month extension to lose weight, and if I didn't, I'd start taking medication, like a good girl. The three months are about to end, and I know that it's irresponsible to go on like this and that this week, I'll have to accept the ultimate label of "diabetic patient" and start taking medication.

At night, we saw a little spark
Bursting from an electric wire.
A bird made an error
And closed a circuit.
Through a limp body
Light shone
In a way, she never dreamt
She could shine.

A weightless, small coal,
A kid bounced it
In the morning
And whistled.

I'm surfing alongside Ayelet without really doing anything special but begin with myself from time to time, but that's not much.

Ayelet Kalter

This can't go on for much longer.

I'll either take action and move forward courageously, or I'll keep doing what I've done most of my adult life about my obesity, which to simply be obese.

I don't need Ayelet for that, and neither does she need me.

But I can't continue sitting on the fence, hanging off this dangerous wire.

I have to get down slowly. Slide down the electric post.

Carefully.

Start walking on the compassionate soil.

If I continue hanging off this wire, one wrong move, and the circuit will end up closing on me.

And without fireworks, there will be nothing but a pile of coal left.

Fragments of eroded sun
Turning in my belly
A washer
That cannot
Get rid of the dirt
(Tamar)

"To be filled from the inside — not the outside."

Tal arrived for therapy about two and a half years ago.
Redheaded.
Diet?! She said.
Not full-on fat, but a few kilograms, she thought, would "put her life in order."
Black, tight leggings, T-shirt with a low neck, Nike shoes, and a timid smile.
A P.E. teacher, ex-athlete, ex-married, ex-happy. Thirty, divorced for about three years. No kids.
Bursting with energy, vibrant.

So, we started like we always do.
Losing weight.
And, as with any beginning, it worked. She cooperated and lost weight. Not too fast, with endless suspicion, but she lost. Four kilograms, and that's it.
It was a bit strange. Because usually in the first "diet round," most people succeed in a losing a lot of weight and fast. They are mostly driven by ambition to succeed in the new project.

In many cases, the newness of it has a constructive, catalytic effect. The problems begin in more advanced stages.

But here? A month or two, and that's it. Four kilograms only.

And she's been floundering ever since. Trying to lose, touching "slimness" and running away. Eating a lot, enjoying the food, occupied with it, taking pleasure in it, loving it.

During our long dialogue, I felt that she was ready to understand that therapeutic success doesn't have to be reaching the ideal slimness of 52 Kgs. She gave up the "perfect." She was willing to accept herself as fleshy to some degree, as she put it. That is, if you're calling out numbers, she'd love to drop 6 Kgs., down to 62. But even there, she finds it hard to reach.

If we look at the two and a half years we've known each other, two major things happened. She isn't as thin as she fantasizes, but she feels and knows how to accept herself the way she is. She knows she can find a partner even at her current weight. What's more, she's less preoccupied with weight as the number on the scale.

So where are we at in the process? Or where do we actually want to get to? If slimness, defined as the ideal weight, is no longer her aspiration in life, and she knows and likes herself the way she is, why not give up this struggle entirely and simply live day to day without endless attempts to lose weight and frustration?

Tal was a professional athlete who has struggled with excess weight her entire life. She has always felt she wasn't thin enough. There was always something to improve as she strived for perfection. Not one extra morsel, everything shows and thus is forbidden. Tal was desperately captive in her desire to be the best, perfect, obsessed with every extra kilogram added to her body and every bite she dared enjoy.

As an adult, she went to study at Wingate.[30] And there, too, the obsessive preoccupation with body, good, and image. She carried on a life similar to that of many others, a routine of studies, love, partnership, and dieting.

And the diet, like some hump, was present all the time. What characterized the "then" hump was Tal's ability to live with it by her side. Whereas today, not only did the hump grow, but it has also taken on some important roles in Tal's life.

What happened in her life that shuffled the status quo between herself and her body? I think Tal's romantic life is partially a mirror of the relationships in her life. Most of them are close relationships, based on Tal's ability to boundlessly care for her partner or friend. She makes sure to be attentive to the other's needs and satisfy them consistently. She diminishes her needs and is busy finding favor and pleasing.

---

[30]Israel's National Centre for Physical Education and Sport was named in honor of British Major General Orde Charles Wingate.

With romantic relationships, it's stronger than ever. She lives in complete symbiosis.

There is no Tal. There is only Ohad. His needs, his desires.

The same goes for the weight.

Ohad watched her, or better yet, she watched her weight for him. Everything about it was for him. And where was she for herself?

Ohad and Tal divorced.

The solitude, aside from being a total shocker, was something she wasn't familiar with. Frightening and consuming. It threatened her entire being. It created a huge void, an endless abyss. A vacuum.

The divorce came out of the blue for her. Just like that. No precursor, no signs. A fact.

It all began with her difficulty conceiving. Tests, basal charting, some hormones for reinforcement. At the same time, Ohad cheated on her. And the more hardship accompanied the attempts to conceive, the more frequent his infidelities became. When she finally achieved a healthy pregnancy, she had to abort it because their relationship deteriorated all at once.

And he left.

She remained alone.

What did she know? No one prepared her for such a life story.

No one told her that solitude is vulnerable, terrifying.

For Tal, the partnership was a huge togetherness. There, in that togetherness, she had no room for herself.

And suddenly, she is on her own.

And she gained weight.

Ten kilograms, which is a lot for her.

There was no one left to be thin for.

Someone had to watch over her, and since she was alone, who would do that for her?

She never took care of herself.

Two old antagonists came back into Tal's life: the food and the fat. One cannot exist without the other; one feeds off the other. Together, they became her companions, tied to her in an amazing symbiotic duo. She's no longer alone; they're with her, watching her steps, hiding her from herself, from others.

And so, she remained in this new, unfamiliar aloneness. A little different, a little heavier.

But very much present.

What do you do with this aloneness?

Escape it.

Go out all the time. Friends, restaurants, entertainment to no end. Just so as not to know, not to feel.

And the food is there, too. A restaurant for lunch, a restaurant for dinner. Countless calories. And Tal loves to eat and indulge in the sheer pleasure of eating.

A day could start with two slices of bread at home, with cheese or chocolate spread. But that was it for banality.

Lunch met her at the café, where she couldn't leave without a decent pasta dish and a hot chocolate fudge cake. And if that weren't enough, nighttime would lure her into new gastronomic temptations. She would sip cappuccino along with a toasted bagel with yellow cheese and Halvah parfait for dessert. And so, another average day would end with at least 2,200 calories. And a little extra fat on.

She's out nearly every evening. Running from herself, wasting calories and gaining weight. She's on a roll. Constantly active. Anything but to be alone with herself.

Throughout our therapeutic journey, Tal seems to have come a long way in accepting herself the way she is. Yes, she would like to be thinner, but slimness had become somewhat less of a pressure point in her life. She has learned to love herself and accept herself for what she is. She realized and felt that she can be loved without having to be thin.

So why not give up this preoccupation with weight and slimness? What is so frightening about giving up the will to be thin?

When we began to touch on it in depth, we discovered that in her mind, a romantic relationship was only possible if she were thin. A thin Tal is a Tal a partner can be with and have room. So long as the fat is there, it doesn't allow for anyone else to join the union, so to speak. It's either Tal with the fat or Tal with a partner.

And she remains fat.

And the food? It controls her, just like Ohad did.

Partnership is a wonderful thing, but dependency is a different story. A painful one.

"What have you gained for yourself by adding fat to your body?" I asked.

"Security," she said, "but also a lot of sensuality and pleasure in eating, and mainly a topic to obsess over—dieting, a topic with which I can fill every possible void. By giving up dieting, I may not only give up being thin but also be left with a void. Ever since Ohad left me, I've noticed that my preoccupation with food and dieting fills some nagging void that is digging at me."

I thought that if she managed to develop a self that would be hers only—not borrowed or reliant but independent and uniquely hers—perhaps she would be able to give up the fat. A self that perhaps she could love. She looked at me reluctantly and chuckled. "Self?" she asked. "How will I know who that 'self' is? I don't even know it. I don't even know where I could find it; I don't think it exists in me. I'm so used to experiencing myself through others."

"What happens in your interpersonal relationships?" I asked.

She thought for a moment, looked at me somewhat shyly and said in embarrassment, "I find it hard to believe that what I have inside is worthwhile, valued and real. Even though it's solely mine, I've always been preoccupied with what others want to find in there instead of what I could really be."

"That's draining," I said.

"Constantly being attentive to other's needs, their thoughts, expectations of you, their wishes. It's hard to tell and perhaps even impossible," I added.

The men Tal has met since separating from her husband were very self-centered, and Tal was busy giving, pleasing.

One of them would throw at her, "Look at yourself, it won't hurt you to lose a few kilos!" And Tal would hear and let it slide. She didn't dare wonder if she felt good in the relationship; she was busy trying to please her partner. She tried to enjoy trips to the Judea desert, the small things. But she wasn't really satisfied. She didn't really love.

But she didn't leave either, she didn't choose for herself. Until they chose for her and left.

The same thing happened to her with Yair, handsome, charming, with an impressive social status, but that's it. I remember how she told me she would arrive at his house, and he would be glued to the TV, staring into it. There was no conversation, no interest on his part, and not much of a physical touch either. But Tal didn't leave. Despite her feelings of hurt and humiliation, she stayed the night. And in the morning, as she escaped, she realized what she has done to herself. How in her fears and insecurity, she plants herself in situations that hurt her.

I believe she has reached a point and a recognition that instead of looking for herself in foreign fields, she must remain with herself a little and discuss, understand, feel and know. What happened there, in Ohad's abandonment? What is this solitude? What was she hurt by, and what is she so afraid of?

I was wondering when she would give up her strong dependency on the other and discover her own reservoirs inside her. Will she be able to desire for herself? And perhaps, she can make room for someone to live at her side, instead of living for him. And then, maybe she can give up the fat in her life.

A year later.

"To be filled from the inside, not the outside."

These are no longer foreign words.

She can feel them. She knows who she is.

She dares to feel all of her inside, and the void isn't filled by a substitute partner or by shedding the expected kilograms.

The void is there, but it no longer consumes her.

She knows her value and believes in it. It is no longer measured by her weight.

It is measured from inside her; not by being thin or fat.

It is measured by her ability to see herself for what she is, acknowledge herself as an independent, separate being.

Not as part of…

And she? She continues to look wonderful even without dropping weight. She is successfully studying for her master's degree and continues to run a flourishing sports center.

And most importantly, she owns herself fully.

For me it's wonderful.

I know it's the same for her.

December 5, 2001

Still, despite it all, with the tiny steps I take back and forth, I lost weight.

Not much, but I reached a new, lower weight, a weight I haven't been in for a long time. The most important thing is that clothes that haven't fit me for maybe four years are fitting me.

I have a few wardrobes in my closet.

A line of clothing that fits me, and I feel relatively comfortable in because they're big enough. They don't cling to my body.

The kind that make you feel like you're an invisible fat person. A feeling only meant for fools. And I have another line of clothing that is slightly smaller by a size or two, which I wear when I lose 5–10 Kgs.

I feel pretty comfortable in them.

Comfortable, a purely relative word.

You never truly feel comfortable with such a big body.

And of course, there are the clothes that I've been saving for a long time, and they move from season to season, summer and winter.

Those are the closet clothes.

The fantasy clothes.

Those that fit me once. Each year, slowly but surely, I give away cloth and after cloth. So as not to let go of the fantasy all at once.

Enjoy the moment.

Enjoy what there is now.

Enjoy the pants you haven't worn in four years.

December 6, 2001

And I, who takes pleasure in the written word gushing out of me? I was dried up.

And I, who feeds on crowded rows of words?

I lost most of the songs that I wrote in the last year and a half.

Dozens of precious poems swallowed in the computer's bowels.

How did it dare to devour them like that, without leaving a trace?

The poems contained bitterness and sadness, pain for the loss of innocence. They depicted the disillusionment at the belief that I could lead my patients to a safe haven. I think I became more realistic and as such, more calm and accepting.

I lost some of myself, some of that infinite power that burns inside me, and a lot of the determination and faith.

Something in my eternal flame cracked.

Something in my turbo engine eroded.

How is that related to you, Tamar?

I'm tired.

I didn't just stop writing or three months and let you wallow in the bog you created for yourself.

I'm tired of fighting for you, pleasing you, worrying about your health, smiling.

I'm tired.

Less goading, less supportive, less able to conjure energy from within myself to give to you. Indeed, I'm here with you, committed, but tired.

I'm tired of the endless talk about insights and realizations. Of accepting.

Yes, you made it down to a new weight yesterday. You were excited. I saw that. I think you lost an entire kilogram. Nothing thrilling.

But symbolically, it was a big and significant step for you. I'm leery of celebrating. Everything is so fragile and slippery. But you, you smiled like I haven't seen in a long time. You radiated joy. For you, this kilogram was a shift, a small progress. And you rejoiced in it. About two weeks ago, we tried to dig within you, to search. We know that your ability to lose weight depends on your willingness to give up the "odd" roles you have given the fat without even realizing it. You're not one of those women who must fast in order to lose weight. You don't have to eat 800 calories a day. It's enough if you cut back on quantities, eat less fatty food, and the change will take place for you to lose weight. But, even this action, which seems so easy, you have a hard time implementing.

This brings us back to your ability to understand the essence of what the fat is to you, the playing between life and death. Your ability to reach the edge and only there get a fright and take a step back. But only one step. You keep smelling the danger, the burning of adrenaline in your veins exploding with fat. We went back to ancient times when you would go wild without limits. Your wild relationships with men and violent motorcycle races. You would hit the brake on playing with fire only when your feet got scorched. Only when you felt threatened.

And today?

The same thing, only undercover. You rampage your body with great intensity.

Not just fat; humungous fat. Not just ailments, high blood pressure, raging diabetes, cancer. Terminal illnesses, not pretend ones, not as if, real. And every time, you gather yourself right on the threshold a minute before you crash.

You take tests to calm down. Only then do you touch yourself, but even then it's "as if." You get a fright for two to three weeks, feign struggling, and after a while, you disappear with your tail between your legs.

And so forth.

And so, today, as in the past, your life is mixed with storms and sweeping draughts full of excitement and surprise. Back then, they were innocence death games, and today they are life games for real.

An event!

Yes, it indeed calls for mentioning. For the first time since we began our joint journey, you feel like you've lost weight in so as it allows you to wear clothes you haven't worn for years.

Yes. I see your excitement. I tend to get carried away in the childish whim that takes over you, but am careful. Everything is temperamental, extreme, and slippery. Despite that, I try to enjoy the here and now, not develop expectations, not be preoccupied with what's next, be with you in this wonderful place you so wanted to get to. A place which is seemingly a small step, but for you, it harbors hope, light. Corduroy pants in all kinds of colors, a desire to try on clothes, to stand in front of the mirror. And it's only one kilogram. But it's a lot in a sea of endless stagnancy, it's the feeling and knowledge that something is happening.

I'm with you, Tamar. I'm for you.

December 15, 2001

Aye...you're tired.

I see it in you without you having to write about it.

I see you continue doing a lot, as you're used to, but with very little joy. Very little festivity. Very little excitement.

I see you exhaust every topic really fast, rushing to move on. You're not really able to be or snuggle into your infinite doing.

How tiring this is, Aye.

What tires me the most are your transitions from topic to topic.

You can't stay with anything for more than a moment.

You know in a flash what's there, how you feel, what the person before you is about to say and feel. How predictable, how boring, how dull. There is no power to the experience.

And our areas of overlap are so few because each one is entrenched in herself. And that's something new to you, Aye.

I know you're suffering from back pain. I see it in your paleness, the sitting angle on the chair, the movement of your head. And your physical, worrying, frightening, threatening pain of your betraying back annoys you. So much! Or is that what you're willing to put out to me—annoying?

In addition, perhaps, you're falling apart from the inside, but you can't touch it, or it will crumble you. You protect yourself well against me, making sure to switch as soon as I respond too intimately. You know your games are getting on my nerves. I'm not sure I can continue this journey like you wanted and planned.

Who defines ahead of time that you remain the therapist throughout?

You also know how to play, Ayelet.

In your restrained way, you play with the boundaries, and I'm not really interested in staying exactly there.

Intimacy is one-directional, fucked up, phony, non-existent. I don't want it like that anymore.

I don't want you jumping from topic to topic in one second.

And you can be with me, Ayelet, really, if you only be yourself.

I don't want to give into you like this anymore.

You know more about me than anyone else around me.

You know so much about my life. About me.

I don't want to give that to you anymore. I don't want to give myself anymore.

It's too big of a present.

And you, inside your nook, in your Perspex bell, with your strong, aligned spine.

It can relax a little, your spine if you only give it some air and space and not confine it so strongly. I don't want to give myself to you anymore under these terms.

Open yourself up a little, bring your fatigue. Maybe we can be tired together. You want me? Then compromise. Not for me, for yourself. You will gain me. Give me something else. Give me some of you. Maybe that will stir us.

Aye...I'm tired.
I don't run like you.
I'm also crushed, like the crushed vertebrae in your scrawny body.
I don't want to give you my insides anymore. It drains me.
Unless you come to me with a little more than the predictable story of the therapist and the patient, I won't do it anymore.
You're meaningful to me.
It scares me, shuts me down, and I don't want it in these terms anymore.

Tell me something about yourself, Aye.
I'm like you, so tired. For me to be, is to be how I am with food.
The way I eat is part of who I am, just like I breathe, I suck it into me in the quantities I've gotten used to.
It's part of my existence. Like any other daily physical action. Shower, dress, sleep. In order not to eat food the way I eat it, I must make an effort, be aware and in control. All the time. And I'm tired.
I'm tired of my demanding job. I must be available and free, and at my best, and under a magnifying glass, and an object, and a leader who's constantly being tested. It's so exhausting and draining.
Now I don't have the strength for anything.
The little I have left, I try to give to the kids and Nadav, for whom I've had nothing left to give lately.

December 26, 2001

And perhaps I am your mirror, and through me, you express anger at yourself?

Am I the only one running?

Maybe I look like a spin top, circling in endless movement.

And you, Tamar? Are you resting? As if.

Simply because you're heavier and it's harder for you to get around. You're motivated by ongoing restlessness, a relentless inner drive. Nadav and the kids are your anchor to reality; they connect you back to the ground that is shaking under your feet, threatening to swallow you at any minute.

Nadav in his serenity, his regular job, his ability to listen to you without getting anxious, absorbing all your idiosyncrasies. Like running in the middle of the night to bring you a CD without which you cannot start an event. So, with patience and love, he illustrated your business cards, sitting at the computer for hours printing them for you. Every day, he makes you sandwiches for work, hoping this will help you watch your food intake. He even does healing and reflexology treatments on you, to relax your body.

And the kids.

Different from you.

Your eldest daughter maintains a tranquility that you envy. You envy her way of accepting things, her mature, forgiving way of viewing the world around her. But I think you envy her very being. A curious adolescent, guzzling the world.

And your son, introverted and reclusive but radiating power and strength. As you like it.

Their existence in your life protects you.

And what protects you here, with me?

Do you truly believe that if I remove the boundaries, I can continue to be your therapist?

Do I have to bring myself as a patient only because you do?

Perhaps the sense of closeness and intimacy in the sessions enables reciprocity? I think we've become a little enmeshed in each other.

And besides, Tamar, perhaps what you're sensing is a different relationship from the one you're used to.

Usually, you're in the role that I'm currently playing in your life. I, not you is the one who seemingly has power. I'm the giver, and you're the receiver. This is not a familiar position for you, nor do you feel comfortable in it. And you try to gravitate our dynamic to a more familiar place by reversing the roles. Perhaps this is part of your lesson here.

And I, Tamar, make sure to be present, so that a pleasant feeling reigns between us, but to a certain extent so that I don't become the patient. I share situations with my patients that I believe may help them.

For instance, most of the people ask me, "How can you understand us if you don't even suffer from being overweight?" And I share with them that I, too, have a tendency to gain weight, and I also share the love of food, for which my genetics doesn't really help.

Or when they ask me about the eating habits at my house, I tend to give them a general picture, so that the patient can learn about me, even if a little. I tell them about a house where we eat everything: vegetables and oats but also junk. Because that's how it is when you choose to be in the middle rather than any extreme. Within this middle, I try to impart to my children a different way of thinking about prioritizing foods—healthy and less healthy—and how to enjoy food as entertainment, too.

I find that this sharing brings us closer, which makes me a tangible person that can be trusted. Because my house, too, faces a challenge with junk food and a tendency toward obesity. And there isn't always healthy food cooked ready.

But this sharing, Tamar, is only part of the therapy, not beyond it.

Could it be that your anger toward me is because you feel I kept myself outside?

Tamar, you don't even know how far deep I am. Deep, loving, wanting. So what if I don't show it all? So what if I don't say and you don't exactly know?

And you answered, in your gentle, unique way, "I don't understand, Ayelet, I'm not complaining. On the contrary. I'm not angry either. I feel good here, next to you, it's interesting, different. But I want more. More of this Ayelet, who I'm getting to know, and discovering that beneath this personal and therapeutic distance, there are deposits of vitality, empathy, sharpness of mind and originality. I so wanted to taste them, to feel them a little more. But you don't let me. You don't let yourself. And not just because we are patient-therapist. It's more than that. Even in the neighborhood, in social gatherings, you don't mingle easily, you keep a tempting, intriguing distance. But when I draw closer, I want more.

"You're attentive to me, you feel and understand me without me having to explain. By my intonation, expression, the way I stand. You're not deterred by my escapades. You're patient with my hide-and-seek games. You remain strongly rooted. I know you'll understand; you won't accuse or reprimand, and that makes it easier for me. I would have probably escaped without a trace from other places."

December 31, 2001

End of the year.

You missed a session again.

You chose not to show up.

"Just don't be offended," I told myself. "Just don't take it personally."

I immediately worry if I hurt you, or said things I should have kept to myself, like putting up therapeutic boundaries, my inability to share with you what I'm going through as a person.

I really don't know.

How come you asked your secretary to call and cancel the session? Your secretary? Not you? Am I so threatening? Is the fear of confronting me what got you motivated to act remotely? Did the closeness you began to feel quickly push you back out?

And perhaps it's your resistance to therapy. Or to me as the therapist. Is it your way of putting up boundaries? Your way of saying to yourself and to me, "I'm not here"?

I know how hard and painful it is for you. But it's hard for me, too, sometimes, though differently, as the therapist, but hard nonetheless. I take things personally, I get hurt, I have a hard time making separations.

I felt a pinch, but I'm not planning on staying in offended mode for too long. I'll try to be there for you, Tamar, even if remotely.

March 23, 2002

I opened my journal today, curious to see how much time I hadn't written.

It's lying on the floor, in the bedroom, by my side from the first day we started, along with the poem notebook.

The poem notebook got lost.

Now the new poem notebook Ayelet bought me lies there... She wrote, "Love, Ayelet."

I love her too by now.

She also lost her poems. Some of them are typed on her computer.

Mine got lost in oblivion.

How we both lost our words?

Perhaps mine are starting to run out?

I'm out of things to say, to write. And I wanted to move away, and I checked out.

Hollow pearls.
Floating.
An obedient line
Of sand grains
Covered
In a white glare of pain.

May 23, 2002

Tamar, we both took a hiatus. We sank into abysmal fatigue. Somewhat decadent. We lost ourselves. Each one in her own way. Close, yet distant.

I haven't written in five months. Neither did you.

Five months of weltering.

You rarely came to sessions. You rarely brought yourself to face your eating.

And I? Something in me dulled.

I looked at you, at your size, I felt the heaviness, your exhaustion from yourself, and mostly the powerlessness.

I've grown tired of fighting for you.

All I can do is remain in the small space I have left by you.

And you, Tamar, you know me, you feel, but not.

And you, Tamar, you want, but are defeated.

From all the insight and knowledge of yourself, you remain bound by the golden threads you weaved, captive in endless words that shield and touch but never penetrate.

They never penetrate you.

They never penetrate your deposits of fat.

And now, they are left as nothing but testimony.

I ask myself how to utilize the wealth inside you, so it works for you and not against you. And I don't know. Another technique, another introspection, another ailment, all these aren't enough to propel you into separating from the fat and the food.

So you've given up on health, femininity, agility?

You've given up on yourself?

I'm sad, Tamar. And there is not even the slightest hint of my disappointed self here.

I haven't written for weeks, perhaps even months. Neither have you.

Why didn't I write for so long? Maybe because you weren't here for me to write to. Maybe because I wasn't here either, to write to you. The moment I realized you were playing with cards turned over, I too began to fight for you less and less. I got tired of circling in the castrating bog of fat.

The moment you checked out, do did I. It's not simple. To constantly supply nourishing energies without getting feedback. Even a little.

I didn't get any.

At first, the very thought that I gave you power, gave me power. But now, when I see that you don't use my gifting on the one hand, yet I accept you on the other, I also get tired. My gifting may very well be different now, murkier, less energetic.

And you, Tamar, why weren't you present?

Because you don't feel comfortable connecting.

Because it's hard and you give up.

You find countless reasons as to why. But no reason truly convinces you, because you know just as I that they are nothing but thick mist and a blinding sheath, and that is how you've been operating for so many years.

It's hard for me to see you drowning in your sea of fat.

I'm still here. Offering empathy, security, and perseverance. But also sad.

Sad?
Not just for myself.

"The day Betty entered my office, the instant I saw her steering her ponderous two-hundred-fifty-pound, five-foot-two-inch frame toward my trim, high-tech office chair, I knew that a great trial of countertransference was in store for me.

"I have always been repelled by fat women. I find them disgusting: their absurd sidewise waddle, their absence of body contour... I could scarcely think of a single person with whom I less wished to be intimate."[31]

The day Dana walked into my office for the first time, the moment I saw her navigate her body—one-hundred-fifteen-kilograms, hundred-fifty-meters in height—toward the chair in my office, I thought about Yalom's story.

That same day, after Dana left the session in tears, I quickly went back and reread his story, "The Fat Lady," and felt angry.

Not at his honesty. I actually think it wasn't at him, but at myself, at my own judgmental nature. I asked myself if couldn't see a person for what he is, without automatically building him a story, without projecting my feelings, thoughts and pain on him.

---

[31]Yalom, Irvin D. Love's *Executioner: And Other Tales of Psychotherapy*. Basic Books Inc. Publishers, New York, 1989.

I didn't feel disgusted like Yalom. I felt sadness, perhaps pain, but these too, as the feelings of disgust, were not free of criticism.

I ran endless scenarios, built mountains of theories. I decided that Dana was an old, single woman, solitary, with no friends, without a rich cultural world or a life full of interest. The only thing I didn't do was to simply look at Dana in the purest way possible.

A fat woman.

A round face, connected to sagging shoulders as one piece.

A neck drowning in a sea of fat.

A heavy, cumbersome body nestled in soft, colorful fabrics.

Short legs.

And teary eyes.

Fifty years old.

Divorced with two kids.

I ask, she answers. As if she prepared the answers ahead of time. As if she practiced what she would say.

"What do you eat?" I asked.

"I eat shit, other people's shit," she said.

And what do you do with your own "shit" if you eat other people's shit?

"I can't find my own shit because I'm full of other people's," she answered.

And when she's full, she can't think, feel, touch the pain.

"What is there deep inside your body?" I asked. "A hole," she answered.

And added, "Once I thought that the hole was the size of a uterus, and that if I had a baby, the hole would disappear because it would be filled by the baby in my uterus.

"And indeed, I didn't gain weight during my pregnancies that much. Now the hole is like a fist. Maybe a rubber ball. It's in the middle. At the center of the Solar Plexus.

"A black hole.

Once, like I said, the hole was bigger."

"What made it shrink?" I asked.

"Life," she said.

And I asked, "And the obesity?"

"Maybe the bigger I get, the less space the hole has. And then it's less painful, less touching, less feeling," She answered.

"Try to talk to it, to this hole. What does it look like, how does it feel to you?"

It seemed that from the moment the floodgate opened, the words poured out unstoppably.

Dana spoke in English, her native tongue. I chose to quote things as they were said due to their richness of language.

My bulk... my bulk... no one else's I sit here, and don't want to think about it... I force myself to see it. I find it degrading... why do I need this... today... I ate, one sweet roll, with butter, one regular roll with the tuna and corn and... and butter, be honest... last night was good till Rozi came... she ate a roll... and I ate half, with butter... why??

I drank juice. More caloric... why can I not say goodbye to you fat... what do you mean to me?

Warmth, comfort... giving to others.

Why can't I give myself???

I ask myself what is going on... I cannot understand it.

OK, stop understanding, just do it... I find myself confused... what is it about Rozi that makes me eat?... is it her dependency on me that makes me angry?

I give up so much of myself for what reason? Why?? Give up time, precious to me last night... gave up the comfort that I seek, give up work time... my happiness at my success.

Why do I not value my time better, my giving... she comes and takes over, she smokes, she sits in my bed, like a small child, and I give up my soul for her, she say... "I only feel secure when I am near you... do you feel the same?" I say: "no... I feel secure on my own." Is this true? If so, why am I feeling that I need to give myself up when she is here? Why do I lose part of me? Why do I give up my soul? Not just to her, but to so many?

I wonder... such nice news about Paris... it seems they will take me on... I am so flattered.

Paris, to study there, my dream... I wonder where my feelings are. Ray says, Rozi will never give you up for anyone. She needs you to breathe. ...OK... back to me... why did I eat today? Burekas... were not even good ones... why??? Where am I when I eat??? I know Rozi selfish... but where am I???

What is going on... will continue later...

I have been thinking... today is Monday, and I keep thinking that if I lose weight, I will be small, take up no place, have no room for myself, I feel abandoned, alone, small... very small... the bulk makes me feel I have a place, I make room...

***

When I asked Dana to draw the hole, she drew herself as a non-fat woman. This hole inside her was very big compared to her dimensions in the drawing.

In her experience, the more she grows, the smaller the hole becomes, since it has no room. It becomes smaller and smaller until it's hard to feel it.

Dana thought that the pregnancy would fill up the hole since she would be huge anyway, but was let down. She thought a man could do it, but here, too, she was let down. The relationships she created emptied her more than they filled her.

However, when she talks about her daughter, who lives and studies abroad, you can see the light and color in her face. She feels like the hole is filled with trees, flowers, and sun. But this happens so rarely. Most of the time, it's a dark, threatening hole. And she is small, and the hole is big; it ambushes her and threatens to consume her. And the far, like a giant winter coat, covering everything, especially this hole. So, they don't see or know. And then, the fat in all its might swallows the hole into its guts.

She feels like she is being fed all the time, not like she's choosing to eat. "What happens if the shit there, and you manage not to eat it?" I asked.

She finds it difficult to answer.

She cries again.

> I smile and smile
> I won't let them see
> The pain that sits inside of me
> I feel it strong each time I see

The slime that's left inside of me.
I question who is feeding me
This slime that sits for all to see
And then I know
Without a doubt
This is I that forces it down my throat

I wish to vomit, once again
And let to fall... but not on them
Not on any part of man
Because I feel
It's not for them
Man can offer shit to me
It's up to me, for me to see
That shit is bad, it's bad for me.
Refuse I say. Refuse to eat
This stuff that means so much to me
It is not love or caring... see
It is just food wrapped up in thread
Thread of shiny colored dread
Which means nothing once it's fed

Fed to me,
Instead of love

Why accept this role I dread
To swallow shit I am being fed?

I hope to find another way
To swallow only what I may
What makes me feel I am fresh and gay

Still healthy and be able to say
This I who choose, not them by far
I choose who sits here in my heart
I also choose what comes inside my mouth

And lies
Inside my gut
And not the slime
That others chose for me to hide.

***

What happens if you no longer play the victim's role, the one who eats everything he's being fed?" I asked.

"Nothing," she said. "I'm tired," she mumbled.

"I feel like my stomach has been beaten up by all those who wanted to feed me," she said.

"Maybe you should throw up on them?" I tried.

She watched me, scared.

"What will happen to you if you throw up?"

No response.

"And who is 'they'?"

"I think it's Mom and Dad," she said. "Mom would always say, 'You don't count, and your needs should not be considered because you really don't have any,'" she whispered.

Dana is in endless pursuit of love all the time.

She constantly tries to please others, give them what she thinks they want from her. This is how she was raised, to please her parents' needs, so that perhaps, this way, she will earn some moments of grace.

But Dana feels like she gets shit from her environment, swallows it, and returns flowers. She will return flowers even if this gifting hurts her. Sometimes she feels injured by shards of glass that scratch her, and she bleeds but continues to give despite it.

"What about the men in your life?" I asked carefully.

She replied, "I think they like my company. To sit down and talk to me, but never from a sexual place. Not from a desiring, lustful place. Not from passion.

"All the men in my life hurt me. My father was the first one.

I received and felt some of his love for me only when I pleased him.

His love for me was always conditional.

It wasn't a love based on my mere existence as his daughter, but on what I did for him, or how I treated him.

Conditional love.

"I never asked myself what I expected for myself; I was always there just for him.

I think this is a pattern that repeated itself in most of my relationships with the opposite sex.

I would try to give, spoil as much as I could, and so I would lose myself.

And I always remained empty.

There was no one to fill the vacuum that was formed, the void.

And then came the food. It was always there, always within reach, delicious and pleasurfull. I would choose it, as much as I wanted, and it was for me. Only for me. And then there was a lot of food, a lot and alone."

Dana took a deep breath, suppressing a tear and continued.

"When Dad died, I gained twenty kilograms."

"And Mom?" I asked, "where is she in your life's story?"

"My mom hated me because I was pretty. She tried to kill my sexuality. She didn't even buy me a bra when I grew up.

"I was a real beauty," she recalled.

"Mom was jealous, and hurtful. She didn't buy me clothes, she didn't let me pamper myself, she didn't let me express my femininity, she isolated me."

"Like in Snow White?" I asked.

Dana looked at me, silent.

"Why do you choose to remain mommy's girl at the age of fifty?" I asked.

"I think that every reference to my fat takes me back to my childhood, to my mom. In my experience, my mom hurt me throughout my life, and she really continues to do it to this day. I can't separate myself. I'm still there, accepting the verdict.

"I feel like I'm really victimizing myself in my relationship with Mom, with some of my group study colleagues, but mainly with men. You know, it's very apparent in my group study.

"As usual, I try to be liked, but I feel that no matter what I say, my words always elicit negative criticism, as if my fat announces, 'Dana? There is no way she has anything clever to say.'

I feel so distanced. Alone.

"It got to the point where before each class, I would become anxious about what they would say to me that day, how they would treat me and whether they would humiliate me. I felt like I was walking on eggshells, bruised and scared. Something in this encounter would put me in the role of the victim, whose abuse is a form of pleasure for others."

She inhaled deeply, looked at me, searching for compassion, solace, embrace. And I gave. A little, carefully.

"What else happens to you with men?" I asked.

Dana continued, "When you're fat, it's as if sexuality doesn't exist. Who wants a fat woman, whose chin is almost connected to her shoulders? Who would want to even get to know me? Despite what I look like on the outside, I am different on the inside, I have love and joy and a lot of passion, but there are no men. They don't come close. Only because I'm fat. I hate this fat."

I could see and feel her sadness, her bitterness.

It was as if everything was blocked for her. She had been robbed of an entire world of feelings and pleasure just because she was heavy-set, which left her in an endless battle for her true place. A pursuit of belonging, acceptance, recognition, love. A pursuit of another place.

What is that place?

I think it wasn't clear for her either. She had learned to search for it in painful ways that weren't right for her. Her being as huge, but really small. It was as if she were hiding inside the fat.

Only there, she was protected.

"What do you desire for yourself?" I asked.

She looked, tears coming again.

She asked mockingly, "Desire? I don't touch that. I'm not allowed to feel it. I can't do anything with it anyway, because there is no one to listen to it, no one to fulfill my needs, so it's better not to know what my desire is. Better not to feel it."

> You ask me what I feel...
> I say it is a void...
> I fill it with food.
> To make me feel I stand on ground,
> Not up in a plane,
> Not knowing where I go
> But here inside
> I do not know
> So each time there is unknown
> I run for food to feel I see...
> My quest for knowledge is just the same
> To make me feel I know the game
> The emptiness I feel
> Is just the great void
> Left behind
> Without appeal
> Not knowing what
> Not knowing where
> Not knowing how the game will end.

***

I didn't try to throw flowers at Dana's feet.

I didn't try to tell her that the road was clear.

I think I helped her open a window into herself, into the world of her fat, without weaving dreams.

I thought that if I provided a loving, unconditional container for her, I would give her a pleasant, unfamiliar experience. And sometimes that is a lot.

That is how I came to her.

Or at least tried.

During our weekly sessions, we spent most of the time trying to understand the role food played in her life. The food journal she religiously wrote in helped us a great deal. It detailed the types of food she ate, the quantities, and the flavors she preferred. We could see through the journal when she ate a lot, when she coped without food, when she chose it and when it chose her.

Dana began to understand that food filled the immense loneliness and void that gnawed at her soul. She felt it was hard without the food because it substituted feelings of love or friends that she wished she had. She realized that she ate a lot when she felt anger and frustration when she could not express her anger for fear it might hurt another, but most of all, for fear it might make the other hurt her. And that she would definitely not be able to contain or feel.

So she remained fat.

She realized that perhaps right then, she could not give it up or fight it.

I asked myself if there was something soothing about it. The very understanding of what she could demand of herself and what she must let go for now. And maybe it was okay that she was the way she then. Thick and heavy and still eating a lot.

Three months went by. We tried to get down to the root of things and put some order in them. We tried to create a framework within the painful chaos of her life. From those insights, we deduced that one cannot always fight or give up the large quantities of food. Sometimes, it's the right thing to leave the food and fat as-is, since they have no substitute and could not be lived without, at least for the moment.

Dana began to accept the idea that maybe she was okay the way she was right then, fat, heavy and still eating a lot.

She completed her academic year and was about to begin her doctoral studies in Paris. In our last session, she looked happy. Something in her was whole.

She was going away.

A new beginning.

Hope.

May 24, 2002

Be in white.
It will clean you, bring you back
Fix your life.

Be in white.
Bleeding rips will grow webs.
The dough of flesh
Jammed under the nails
I will not leave traces.

Be in white.
Snakes that penetrate the body
Leave hollow pores

You can relieve yourself of the dance party
In the cave of illusions

Be in white
And go on dying

(Tamar)

May 31, 2002

We made a new agreement. No expectation.

Every day, at the end of the day, you are to leave me a message on my voice mail with a laconic report of what you had eaten that day.

As part of your work, you treated a youth with a drug addiction. The treatment included a daily report the youth was forced to give you, several times a day, of his actions and behaviors. Through that youth, you realized that just as he is addicted, you may be an addict of some form or another. And that if it benefits him, perhaps it will benefit you.

I offered to do that for you six months ago. But as usual, any invasion of your boundaries threatened to suffocate you. So you resisted.

And now? It came from you.

You invited me.

The rationale behind it was to make the reporting more immediate. That is, with the daily call, both you and I know if you were there for yourself or not.

Moreover, I thought that while the responsibility for reporting remains yours, the very notion that I'm here, day after day, listening and knowing, would perhaps serve you differently. At least for some time. Just to get back on track.

You have been doing this for four days. Every morning, I hear your voice on my voice mail, describing your eating the previous day.

What, when and how much you ate.

Yesterday, for example, you ate:

Two sandwiches with light bread that Nadav made.

A big salad with two veggie patties at work.

You couldn't hold yourself back and ate hot Spanakopita that just came out fresh from the bakery.

At home, you ate a large baked fish with lots of spinach and yellow beans.

In the evening, you slipped slightly, with four slices of light bread with a spread and a small bag of corn puffs.

I listen, without responding, hoping you will continue reporting to yourself and to me.

June 6, 2002

It seems like our last session was somewhat frightening for you.

You realized I was beginning to talk about ending the journey up to now.

I thought it would be right to start winding down our writing, which mainly dealt with the emotional processes we experienced—yours as the patient and mine as the therapist.

Perhaps from now, it would be wise to focus more on the cognitive-behavioral aspect of eating.

For both of us saw, Tamar, that very often the endless soul searching doesn't necessarily promote you.

I know that losing weight is important to your survival. First off, health-wise. We both know that losing another ten kilograms will bring a significant change to your health, and that is what concerns you most at the moment.

The emotional journey we took has been incredibly important. Without it, you wouldn't have stayed here or dropped the first ten kilograms. But that won't suffice. You want to be healthier and happier. In other words, you want to arrive at your own well-being.

Let's look practicality straight in the eye, losing weight, that's it. Let's cope with the practical challenge, giving up, choosing your daily eating.

June 11, 2002

And you tried.

I almost kissed you yesterday.
Would you believe it?
Me?

I debated whether it was proper from a therapeutic standpoint. And perhaps I was worried I would scare you with my burst of excitement.

We have been together for two years, and for the first time, something major happened. Not on the experiential plane, but on the practical plane. You finally switched a digit. You lost an entire kilogram and dropped down to 109 Kgs.

The last time you were at this weight was four years ago when you were sick. Back then, the weight loss wasn't your choice, but yesterday? It was all yours. Thanks to you and the place you chose to be in.
I almost kissed you yesterday.

I was afraid to invade you, I didn't know if this invasion into your body, into your fat, would distance you. I wasn't sure if a gate has been opened or just a tiny hole in a fortified wall. So, I opted not to enter without permission. I didn't want to feel like I was overstepping my boundaries.

I believe that although I didn't touch you, you felt. I also know that switched back to reality very quickly and asked you, "So....? Do you feel like you can stay there? Not get a fright and ruin everything?"

You didn't quite understand what I was getting at.

"Why would I want to ruin it if I'm so happy with my new weight? How can you even think that I would want to binge now? I just want to lose more and more weight. I have so much hope and optimism now. Aye, do you realize that I'm at a weight I haven't been at for years? Are you aware that this change is a real cause for celebration for me?"

And I, with my experience, know that joy and energies aren't' enough. Binges lurk in the shadows, waiting to destruct. I tried to push away my fear and stay present you with you, Tamar, to celebrate.

I was happy. For both of us.

I knew it would happen. Throughout the week, surprisingly consistent, you called every evening to report what you ate. Every evening, you allowed yourself to see what you put into your huge, tired body. Every evening, you remembered that it's only you and it there. Only you and it can listen to each other and even become friendly. I don't know if this laconic reporting of what you ate is what helped you. But it really doesn't matter. The most important thing is that it happened.

And you saw it was possible.

I looked at you.
Huge and present, as always.

And where was I? Suddenly, it didn't matter at all.

I wasn't preoccupied with my place, with my presence alongside you.

I was fully there, for you.

I'm curious to know where we will go from here.

I am slightly concerned because it's the first time you have arrived at this place by yourself, by choosing to reach it. And I ask myself if you will manage to remain in this new place without running away from it. True. You're still fat, very fat, and no one knows and sees the major step you have taken for yourself. But you know. And that is most important.

Yesterday, when you entered the room, there was a feeling of heaviness, fullness. And then you were surprised by this significant weight loss. But the fact that you've called every evening to report what you ate left me undoubting that you will lose weight. Because though you ate a lot, your responsibility to report reduced the quantities to some degree, without your knowledge.

And so it was. And you lost weight.

We both know that the number you reached is only a number, whereas the place you have reached is so symbolical and different. Switching digits is a milestone for every person and for you, it has a double meaning. Firstly, as you said, you went back to a place you hadn't visited in years—the period of being sick and after giving birth to your eldest. Secondly, after wallowing in yourself for months on end, suddenly something shifted, and you were able to make progress and even lose some weight.

It's exciting.

And indeed you are excited.

And the obvious question is how you will feel in this old-new place? How will you feel knowing that this place for you can be comfortable and one you could stay in without running away?

"Running away?" you asked, "where, why? Aye, where are these thoughts coming from? Why would I want to let go of this amazing place? I feel so good in it.

"I know, you're probably worried because I feel good and happy here. Because as you already know about me, these places tend to scare me and I tend to spoil them.

"But Aye, this time, it's different, you'll see. I'm happy with the feedback, the comments, the compliments. They don't scare me. I'm able to enjoy them without messing them up with uncontrollable binges. I think that the journey I've been through has brought me to this place with a different way of thinking and a more realistic outlook. I don't have fantasies about dramatic breakthroughs, unlike before, now I'm able to sit back and enjoy the little I have earned so far.

"I'm proud of this change. It's mine. I feel good with it. Don't worry, Aye."

August 1, 2002

You have maintained this beautiful weight for a month and a half.

We have been celebrating a "decade festival" for a month and a half.

August 16, 2002

Winter, spring, and summer went by.

With a sensitive nose, you can smell the fall within the humid, heavy summer daze.

Fall and winter are my seasons.

In summer, I'm in a coma. I find it hard to navigate the lumps of haze and heat.

I have no air in summer; I suffocate.

The coolness and foliage do me good; when I sense the smell of fall, I know that the kind coolness will come and wrap my big body. And then there is longing in the air. It's always like that in the fall.

A longing.

I haven't written from spring until the end of summer.

I guess I'm starting to part with the writing. Everything seems like it happened so long ago. My life seems old, blurry. I live them like it was an unimportant memory.

Today is our anniversary—eighteen years.

We calculated that I gained exactly 40 kilograms since the wedding, and Nadav gained exactly 20 kilograms—40 kilograms in eighteen years. The kids laughed and said that we expanded the family from within, that they have a lot of Mom; a lot of Tamar.

And I manage to do so little about it.

August 20, 2002

The taste of tomorrow
Invites you to dance
In the shadow of his God's Sycamore.
That knew you all.
In the night of the flesh
That burnt
His soul,
In drunken roots.
Blood
Greenish,
Rusting
His estrangement.

And what about tomorrow, Tamar, shall we continue?

A little forward, a little backward, shall we remain a little stuck?

As far as kilograms, we're minus ten.

We've been talking about change for a few weeks now. About a certain kind of good-bye. About parting from our writing in our journals, but sticking to the weekly sessions and eating journal.

I noticed you were upset. Just when you are a little more successful, just when you talk about change, now of all times? I tried to illustrate to you that although we can see the buds coming to life, something deep in our process is extinguished and needs power, energy, perhaps renewal.

"Aye," you said, "I'm sad. I'm a little scared, but I feel like something about it is better for me. Almost like a certain relief. To stop digging in myself. To be busy with the challenge itself. To harness the little energy in me for weight loss. Not for deep soul searching, but for action.

"For me, the place we have reached is not bad at all. Think about it—for years I've not been able to reach it myself. I've never been consistent with something for so long. You realize what an achievement this is for me? I lost 10 Kgs. (22 Lbs.) For me, that's a lot. And besides, it means there weren't any major hikes in weight in the last two years.

For me, that is success."

August 30, 2002

Aye, you began talking to me about change.

About ending the writing we shared.

About closing our journals.

Closing the two years I put on paper, and continuing on a different path.

Continue meeting, continue keeping an annoying eating journal, focus less on the "why" and more on the "how," which has held me back more than once, and focus more on the practical, on doing.

Two years ago, you invited me to walk this path with you, a road that was more unknown than known. You suggested I write, and I wrote. I wrote like vomiting. I wrote like I write poetry.

Without thinking, without planning, only when I want to.

Whatever came to me. Like in art. I myself didn't remember what I wrote.

And you suggested we read to each other from time to time, and I was surprised by what I poured onto the page. By the exposure, the acquiescence.

It's not easy for me to close this journal.

It's me there.

My guts are spilled inside these pages.

In the last few months, I didn't connect to myself in depth.

I mainly arrived at our weekly sessions. We got weighed.

I gained two kilograms, I lost two kilograms. I didn't do much with myself. My intensive connection with myself, through the written words, threw me into dark places.

It may be time to let go of these places.

Is it worthwhile to focus on the issue itself, on how to continue this Sisyphean process in which I try to gain a little more health and a little more joy?

I lost 10 fragile, slow kilograms. At first, I thought I needed to lose 40 to feel and look good. I'm not there anymore. I only look at the next ten kilograms. How I will lose them? You can't think so far ahead.

True. I gave up my 40 fantasy. Maybe I'm in a more mature, accepting place now. But I know that I can go further. I know that deep inside.

I've never lasted in a weight loss process for two years. Never.

I always ran away after about six months. And I've tried everything. All the diets in the world.

And here, I stayed despite myself.

Why? Because it's different.

It's different than anything I've had in my twenty-year history of obesity.

It's different because, for the first time, I went inside.

It's different because the entire process here is different.

I know it's the only way for me.

I needed this writing to give birth to the pain and become a little free of it. To stop being so addicted to it.

Or better yet, learn how to live with it.

To live with it, but not be paralyzed by it.

To live with it, but be free to do for myself.

For the clear coping with the daily, technical, concrete challenge.

The challenge of eating itself.

September 5, 2002

Today, two years later, I am glad I invited you on this journey, Tamar.

From the get go, I felt it wouldn't be an ordinary journey, with consistent weight loss in a moderate, organized fashion.

I felt that everything in you was jumbled, the boundaries, the fat, practicality, emotions. I was curious to understand, investigate, and discover your visible eating and your concealed eating. I felt that such fat isn't just the result of overeating, but of passions, desires, and needs that are intensely stirring in you.

I wondered if, by understanding and exposing them, you could bring about change in your behavior, perceptions about food and its role in your life. I feel that despite the hardship, we created a change, we arrived at a new and better place for you.

You feel it too.

I know.

It wasn't easy for me.

Facing you.

Facing the expectations. Yours from me, mine from you and mine of myself.

Opposite the disappointments. Yours from me, mine from you and mine of myself.

Facing the stagnancy.

Facing your ability to read me.

Facing your questions, for which I didn't always have the answers.

Facing your pain, which I couldn't always contain or be around.

Facing my therapeutic powerlessness.

Facing my difficulty in wanting for you but not always succeeding.

Facing my difficulty in feeling you so strongly and having that feeling remain inside me.

Facing your fatigue and sometimes mine.

Facing my ability to be with myself.

Facing the slivers of hope that sometimes shattered into shards.

Facing the notion that it could be different.

Facing your fear to remain alone. Facing your strength.

Facing your weakness.

Facing myself.

Facing you.

September 10, 2002

I haven't given up yet.

I haven't given up my wish to be there.

I haven't given up being healthier, prettier, lighter, kinder to my body.

I won't sink in this warm bog.

I want to continue trying to bring more light into this body.

Grace.

In Lieu of Good-bye

Tamar, I didn't know that my soul would be bound to yours.

For two years, we have been walking cautiously side by side.

Mixing a little and then not.

Two years.

Seemingly, not much has happened, but in fact, so much has.

I feel the need to bring to a close my part in this chapter of our lives.

It is beginning to move in somewhat taxing, exhausting circles.

From the moment we began to discuss change, it's as if everything came into life. You woke up from the stupor you sank into, filled with energy and a desire to lose weight.

Two years.

When I look back, I ask myself where you were and where you are today. On the weight index, the road ahead is still long. You are still enveloped in sticky layers of fat. You haven't given all of them up yet. Only some.

A more allowing window has opened up in you, flowing and mostly not despairing. Something in you continues to

Ayelet Kalter

fight for itself. Perhaps that is the difference? And perhaps this is success? The road is hard, exhausting, taxing.

Two years.

It may seem odd that I chose to present such a heavy-handed, draining, and not always optimistic case study. But it seems it is not a coincidence. Our story is not different from other stories. Optimism sometimes lies in the ability to persevere, remain, be present.

And in that, Tamar, you succeeded.

It's easy to drown in this muddy, boggy world.

It seems very easy to succeed; just abstain from food, give up a little. That's all. But reality is far more complex, of course.

There are many gaps in the world behind fat and weight.

The gap between the fantasies of slimness and looking better, and the sincere difficulty in parting with the layers of fat.

The gap between will and ability to act.

The gap between the pain of a life with fat and overweight and the fear of living without them.

The gap between the ability to sit with ourselves and the reality of running away from ourselves.

Perhaps through this journey into the depth of your guts, Tamar, those around you can stop wondering, understand better and stop arguing. Perhaps they can accept and be there for you in a different way than they have gotten used to or known until now.

I wanted to introduce you, the readers, with the difficulty of being different; with the hardship of living in a judgmental society, which promotes slimness as the status quo of success.

I believe we must not force everyone to live under such rigid decrees of ideal weight and food plans. Not all of us were meant to be "thin."

Not all of us were meant to be restrained or altered. Moreover, not everyone can be controlled. This does not mean that a person suffering from obesity lacks will, lacks abilities, lacks motivation, lacks...lacks...lacks... He is different.

I wanted you to get to know yourself from a difference perspective, Tamar. I thought that through you, others could look at themselves, their eating habits, their self-acceptance, and their ways of coping with their eating behaviors.

Tamar, I hope that getting to know yourself differently will lead you to better places for your body and for your soul, why the two have been on bad terms for so many years.

I tried to give you some tools, insights and a lot of containing and acceptance. And mainly be with you, at your side.

They aren't enough, I know.

And still, Tamar, I shall continue to take the same path, shall continue to be there for you and with you.

If you wish to walk with me, I will be there.

If you wish to continue trying, I will try with you.

And the rest?

Is your choice.

Epilogue

Six months later.
Five more kilograms were shed.
And us?
We are still walking.

Acknowledgements

I believe that writing a book is akin to a train engine departing from its station. Some of the train cars are empty, some are full of passengers.

The train travels down a slope and around the bend.

Passengers get on and off at the stations.

And the train?

It continues.

And I?

Like that train.

Traveling.

The road is hard, long and exhausting.

And the passengers?

They change. Getting on and off.

So for all those who dared getting on my train, thank you.

To Danny, who is always there. His love for me gave me the peacefulness to write.

To my children, Amir, Alon, and Yael, for patiently and forgivingly accepting my lengthy absences.

To my father and mother (Gabi and Ruth Nachumov), for accompanying me throughout on my journey in their genuine, unique way.

To Nachmi Drimer, who, from the moment he laid hands on the book, did wonders with his editing and succeeded, not without effort, to bring out the hidden in me.

To Dafna and Zohar Eshet, for being part of my life.

To Yoram Asheim, for a fascinating shoot day that made its mark among the pages of this book.

To those patients, who had and still have a special place in my world, for allowing me to touch, discover, learn and be in awe each time anew.

To all those who walked and still walk by my side, without whom this book would not materialize: Miki Khan, Etty Hazak, Dina Hoshen, Gali Kamil, Daniella Lehavi, Yael Rosenblum and Tsipi Harel.

And I?
I snuggle up in words and simply say **thank you.**

www.ingramcontent.com/pod-product-compliance
Lightning Source LLC
Chambersburg PA
CBHW060232290526
45789CB00001B/17